**PREGNANCY AND INFANTS:
MEDICAL, PSYCHOLOGICAL AND SOCIAL ISSUES**

ECLAMPSIA

PREVALENCE, RISK FACTORS AND COMPLICATIONS

PREGNANCY AND INFANTS: MEDICAL, PSYCHOLOGICAL AND SOCIAL ISSUES

Additional books and e-books in this series can be found on Nova's website under the Series tab.

PREGNANCY AND INFANTS:
MEDICAL, PSYCHOLOGICAL AND SOCIAL ISSUES

ECLAMPSIA

PREVALENCE, RISK FACTORS AND COMPLICATIONS

SHARON WRIGHT
EDITOR

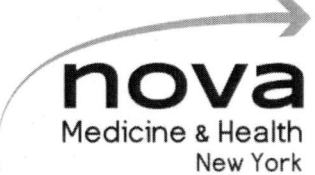

Copyright © 2021 by Nova Science Publishers, Inc.

All rights reserved. No part of this book may be reproduced, stored in a retrieval system or transmitted in any form or by any means: electronic, electrostatic, magnetic, tape, mechanical photocopying, recording or otherwise without the written permission of the Publisher.

We have partnered with Copyright Clearance Center to make it easy for you to obtain permissions to reuse content from this publication. Simply navigate to this publication's page on Nova's website and locate the "Get Permission" button below the title description. This button is linked directly to the title's permission page on copyright.com. Alternatively, you can visit copyright.com and search by title, ISBN, or ISSN.

For further questions about using the service on copyright.com, please contact:
Copyright Clearance Center
Phone: +1-(978) 750-8400   Fax: +1-(978) 750-4470   E-mail: info@copyright.com.

NOTICE TO THE READER

The Publisher has taken reasonable care in the preparation of this book, but makes no expressed or implied warranty of any kind and assumes no responsibility for any errors or omissions. No liability is assumed for incidental or consequential damages in connection with or arising out of information contained in this book. The Publisher shall not be liable for any special, consequential, or exemplary damages resulting, in whole or in part, from the readers' use of, or reliance upon, this material. Any parts of this book based on government reports are so indicated and copyright is claimed for those parts to the extent applicable to compilations of such works.

Independent verification should be sought for any data, advice or recommendations contained in this book. In addition, no responsibility is assumed by the Publisher for any injury and/or damage to persons or property arising from any methods, products, instructions, ideas or otherwise contained in this publication.

This publication is designed to provide accurate and authoritative information with regard to the subject matter covered herein. It is sold with the clear understanding that the Publisher is not engaged in rendering legal or any other professional services. If legal or any other expert assistance is required, the services of a competent person should be sought. FROM A DECLARATION OF PARTICIPANTS JOINTLY ADOPTED BY A COMMITTEE OF THE AMERICAN BAR ASSOCIATION AND A COMMITTEE OF PUBLISHERS.

Additional color graphics may be available in the e-book version of this book.

Library of Congress Cataloging-in-Publication Data

ISBN: 978-1-53619-574-3

Published by Nova Science Publishers, Inc. † New York

CONTENTS

Preface		vii
Chapter 1	Neurological Complications of Eclampsia *R. B. P. Thangappah, K. V. Rajasekhar and S. Baby Vasumathi*	1
Chapter 2	Pre-Eclampsia: It's All About Potassium *Fred Chasalow*	63
Chapter 3	Postpartum Pre-Eclampsia *Igor Lakhno and Kemine Uzel*	115
Index		129

PREFACE

This book is composed of three chapters about eclampsia, which is a condition involving seizures that occur during a woman's pregnancy or shortly after giving birth. Chapter one analyses the clinical profile, neurological manifestations, imaging features, prognosis and risk factors which can predict neurological complications in eclampsia patients. Chapter two describes the discovery of phosphoester steroid conjugates and proposes a role for them in pre-eclampsia. Chapter three discusses postpartum eclampsia and describes which medications should be used for management of symptoms in patients who show signs of pre-eclampsia.

Chapter 1 - Objectives: This study was undertaken to analyse the clinical profile, neurological manifestations, imaging features, prognosis and risk factors which can predict neurological complications in eclampsia patients. Methodology: This retrospective case control study was conducted at Govt. Hospital for Women and Children, Chennai and Meenakshi Medical College Hospital, Kancheepuram from January 2010 to December 2017. During the above period there were 104,989 deliveries and 11,817 (11.3%) were diagnosed with pre-eclampsia and 902 women (0.86%) were diagnosed with eclampsia. The data base identified 76 patients who developed neurological complications and blindness in association with eclampsia. Their case records were analysed for clinical profile, neuro imaging findings and prognosis. Univariate and multivariate analyses were carried out to identify the risk factors for the development of neurological complications and blindness. Results: 8.4% of eclamptic patients developed focal neurological deficits and blindness. The mean age of presentation was 24.91 ± 5.47 years and 57.9% were first time pregnant or delivered mothers. Seizures and neurological manifestations occurred in the antepartum and intrapartum period in 56.6% and in the postpartum period in 43.4% patients. Three patients had atypical presentation. The mean systolic BP was 166.89 ± 24.95 and the systolic BP was >180 mm of Hg in 23.7% of cases. The mean diastolic BP was 114.83 ± 16.34 and the range was between 80-170 mm of Hg. 88.2% showed significant proteinuria. 53.9% of patients suffered from anaemia, APLA and GDM in 3 cases each and HELLP syndrome was seen in 6 patients. Neurological complications noted were hemiparesis/hemiplegia in 57.9% of cases and facial palsy in 21.1% of cases. Aphasia was present in 14.5% and ophthalmoparesis in 3.9% cases. Cortical blindness was noted in 22 patients (28.9%) and in 3 patients there was blindness due to retinal detachment. Imaging studies showed arterial infarcts in 23 patients, intracerebral haemorrhage in 10 patients, CVT and PRES in 8 cases each. The case fatality rate was 14.5% primarily due to cerebral haemorrhage. Conclusion: 8.4% of eclampsia cases developed neurological complications. Postpartum eclampsia, diastolic blood pressure and multigravida were identified as independent risk factors for the occurrence of neurological manifestations in eclampsia.

Chapter 2 - Pre-eclampsia is a risk factor for life-threatening hypertension during pregnancy. Although the symptoms of pre-eclampsia are well known, their underlying biochemistry is not understood. This chapter describes the discovery of phosphoester steroid conjugates and proposes a role for them in pre-eclampsia. The newly discovered steroids are unique in two ways: (a) each steroid is a phosphoester and (b) each steroid has more than 21 carbon atoms. Prior to this discovery, no steroids were known with either feature. None of the newly discovered steroids bind to nuclear receptors. Some of the newly discovered hormones are spiral lactones and function as potassium sparing hormones, just like spironolactone or digoxin. The authors propose that spiral steroids have a key role in pre-eclampsia and may account for the increased, long-term risk of renal and cardiac diseases in affected patients. This chapter has four parts: (a) isolation, structure, and biosynthesis, (b) evidence for function, (c) biological role and function during pregnancy and (d) proposes how the spiral lactones lead to life-threatening hypertension and to the long-term consequences of pre-eclampsia.

Chapter 3 - Pre-eclampsia occurs only in humans during the second half of pregnancy or the postpartum period. It is known to be featured by the development of arterial hypertension and multiple organ failure. The main role of the placental lesions in the pathogenetic scenario was shown. The high level of perinatal pathology is a reason for the continual search in the field. Almost a third of eclampsia occurs in the postpartum period. The pre-eclamptic patients require thorough monitoring of blood pressure and administration of antihypertensive drugs in the puerperium. The pathogenesis and the management of the developed de novo postpartum pre-eclampsia have not been sufficiently studied. The greatest risk of brain stroke after delivery remains for 10 days. It is very important to start the antihypertensives in time. „First-line" drugs should be used not later than 30 - 60 minutes from the time of severe pre-eclampsia diagnosing to prevent intracranial hemorrhage. Labetalol or hydralazine should be used to reduce blood pressure. Sublingual administration of nifedipine may also be considered as „first-line" therapy. The use of magnesium sulfate is necessary for the prevention of seizures in patients with severe pre-eclampsia. In the case of eclampsia, a solution of magnesium sulfate is being administered intravenously at a loading dose of 4 - 5g for 15 - 20 minutes and then the infusion is being continued at a dose of 1 g per hour throughout the day. Uterine curettage is also a possible intervention for reducing blood pressure in women with pre-eclampsia. The clinical case of a systemic inflammatory response syndrome that occurred in a postpartum woman with mild pre-eclampsia is given. Postpartum endometritis, which was caused by group B streptococcus, should have played a triggering role in the progression of preeclampsia. The problem of poly chemical resistance has led to the inability of traditional antimicrobial agents to prevent the dissemination of infection after curettage. The systemic inflammatory response syndrome has contributed to the increased severity of preeclampsia and the development of multiple organ failure.

In: Eclampsia
Editor: Sharon Wright
ISBN: 978-1-53619-574-3
© 2021 Nova Science Publishers, Inc.

Chapter 1

NEUROLOGICAL COMPLICATIONS OF ECLAMPSIA

R. B. P. Thangappah[1,*], MD, PhD, K. V. Rajasekhar[2], MD and S. Baby Vasumathi[3], MD

[1]Department of Obstetrics and Gynaecology,
Government Hospital for Women and Children, Chennai, India
and Meenakshi Medical College Hospital and Research Institute,
Kancheepuram, India
[2]Department of Radiology, Meenakshi Medical College Hospital
and Research Institute, Kancheepuram, India
[3]Department of Obstetrics and Gynaecology,
Government Hospital for Women and Children, Chennai, India

ABSTRACT

Objectives

This study was undertaken to analyse the clinical profile, neurological manifestations, imaging features, prognosis and risk factors which can predict neurological complications in eclampsia patients.

---

* Corresponding Author's E-mail: radhaprabhu54@ymail.com.

Methodology

This retrospective case control study was conducted at Govt. Hospital for Women and Children, Chennai and Meenakshi Medical College Hospital, Kancheepuram from January 2010 to December 2017. During the above period there were 104,989 deliveries and 11,817 (11.3%) were diagnosed with pre-eclampsia and 902 women (0.86%) were diagnosed with eclampsia. The data base identified 76 patients who developed neurological complications and blindness in association with eclampsia. Their case records were analysed for clinical profile, neuro imaging findings and prognosis. Univariate and multivariate analyses were carried out to identify the risk factors for the development of neurological complications and blindness.

Results

8.4% of eclamptic patients developed focal neurological deficits and blindness. The mean age of presentation was 24.91 ± 5.47 years and 57.9% were first time pregnant or delivered mothers. Seizures and neurological manifestations occurred in the antepartum and intrapartum period in 56.6% and in the postpartum period in 43.4% patients. Three patients had atypical presentation. The mean systolic BP was 166.89 ± 24.95 and the systolic BP was >180 mm of Hg in 23.7% of cases. The mean diastolic BP was 114.83 ± 16.34 and the range was between 80-170 mm of Hg. 88.2% showed significant proteinuria. 53.9% of patients suffered from anaemia, APLA and GDM in 3 cases each and HELLP syndrome was seen in 6 patients. Neurological complications noted were hemiparesis/hemiplegia in 57.9% of cases and facial palsy in 21.1% of cases. Aphasia was present in 14.5% and ophthalmoparesis in 3.9% cases. Cortical blindness was noted in 22 patients (28.9%) and in 3 patients there was blindness due to retinal detachment. Imaging studies showed arterial infarcts in 23 patients, intracerebral haemorrhage in 10 patients, CVT and PRES in 8 cases each. The case fatality rate was 14.5% primarily due to cerebral haemorrhage.

Conclusion

8.4% of eclampsia cases developed neurological complications. Postpartum eclampsia, diastolic blood pressure and multigravida were identified as independent risk factors for the occurrence of neurological manifestations in eclampsia.

Keywords: eclampsia, neurological complications, stroke, blindness, risk factors

INTRODUCTION

Eclampsia is an obstetric emergency. It is a potentially life threatening complication of pregnancy characterized by the occurrence of new onset tonic clonic seizures, and/or coma during pregnancy, labour, or puerperium. In 80% to 90% of cases eclampsia is preceded by pre-eclampsia. However, in a smaller proportion of cases, the presentation of eclampsia is atypical and the classical signs of pre-eclampsia, hypertension and proteinuria may not be present. Historically, it was felt that eclampsia represented a progression of the clinical syndrome from pre-eclampsia to eclampsia. But more recent opinion suggests that eclampsia can manifest without prior history of pre-eclampsia, particularly in the late postpartum period [1]. The term "atypical preeclampsia-eclampsia" has been used to describe non-classical forms of hypertensive disorders arising during pregnancy" where the timing of eclampsia may be before 20 weeks of gestation or may manifest 48 hours after delivery or the classical signs of hypertension or proteinuria may not be present [2, 3]. Globally, 42,000 deaths occur every year due to hypertensive disorders of pregnancy which accounts for 14% of all maternal deaths [4, 5]. It has been shown that nearly all of these deaths occur in low-resource settings (99%), with death in high-income settings being very rare [6]. Eclampsia related complications which lead to significant maternal morbidity and mortality are cerebro -vascular accidents (CVA), pulmonary oedema, renal failure, HELLP (haemolysis, elevated liver enzyme, and low platelet count) syndrome, DIC (Disseminated Intravascular Coagulation) and hepatic failure [7]. Studies have shown that in low resource settings, where intensive care facilities are inadequate, pulmonary oedema is the leading cause of maternal death in eclampsia [8], whereas in developed countries, the most common cause of death in eclampsia is CVA [9, 10].

The neurological manifestations of eclampsia include headache, confusion, visual disturbances, blindness, loss of consciousness and stroke leading to neurological deficits. These neurological manifestations are due to cerebral vasospasm and failure of auto regulation of cerebral circulation resulting in hyper perfusion and oedema. The maternal cerebral vasculature is highly vulnerable to adverse effects of preeclampsia/eclampsia. It is associated with increased blood-brain barrier permeability, impaired cerebral autoregulation, hypercoagulability, and inflammation, resulting in complications such as ischemic and hemorrhagic stroke, posterior reversible encephalopathy syndrome (PRES), reversible cerebral vasoconstriction syndrome (RCVS), and cerebral venous sinus thrombosis (CVT). Long-term effects of pre-eclampsia syndrome are cerebral small vessel disease and vascular dementia [11]. The risk of acute cerebrovascular disease in pregnancies complicated by preeclampsia is as high as 1 in 500 deliveries [12]. This study was undertaken to analyse the clinical profile, neurological manifestations, imaging features, prognosis and the risk factors which can predict neurological complications in eclampsia patients.

METHODOLOGY

This was a retrospective case control study conducted at the Government Hospital for Women and Children, Chennai and Meenakshi Medical College Hospital, Kancheepuram, India. The Government Hospital for women and Children is the largest tertiary care maternity hospital in the metropolitan city of Chennai, India and Meenakshi Medical College Hospital is a tertiary care hospital located 70 km from Chennai in the suburban area. The hospitals accept referrals from private clinics, corporation hospitals, maternity/nursing homes, and other primary and secondary care government hospitals. This study was conducted for a period of 8 years from January 2010 to December 2017 after obtaining approval from the institutional review board.

During the above period there were 104,989 deliveries, 11,817 (11.3%) were diagnosed with pre-eclampsia and 902 women (0.86%) were diagnosed with eclampsia. The diagnosis of eclampsia was made based on the occurrence of new onset seizures with generalised tonic clonic convulsions and/or coma during pregnancy, labour, or after childbirth up to 42 days. Though 42 days was taken as the postpartum cut off, all cases were presented within 14 days after delivery. Only those cases fulfilling the criteria for the diagnosis of eclampsia were included in this study. Those women with known seizure disorders and those with pre-existing neurological conditions were excluded from the study. Among the 902 eclampsia cases, the database identified 76 patients who presented with neurological manifestations and blindness in association with eclampsia. The neurological manifestations due to eclampsia included hemiplegia, hemiparesis, facial palsy, aphasia and ophthalmoparesis. The visual disturbances included blindness due to cortical blindness and retinal detachment. 195 consecutive case records of eclamptic women who did not develop neurological deficits/blindness were taken as controls. Stroke was diagnosed according to the definition of the WHO. The World Health Organization (WHO) defines stroke as "rapidly developing clinical signs of focal (or global) disturbance of cerebral function, with symptoms lasting 24 hours or longer or leading to death, with no apparent cause other than vascular origin" [13]. A diagnosis of cortical blindness was made in the presence of intact pupillary light reflexes, intact ocular movements, and normal ophthalmologic findings, thus excluding a peripheral cause of blindness [14]. Retinal detachment was diagnosed at the time of a fundoscopic examination.

Their case records were analysed for the following details: age, parity, period of gestation at presentation, timing of eclampsia, number of seizures, level of consciousness, fits to admission interval, type of neurological deficit, maximum systolic and diastolic BP recorded, preceding symptoms and their duration, medical, obstetrical and eclampsia related complications, severity of proteinuria, fundus changes, investigation results, neuro imaging findings, time interval between fits to delivery in antepartum and intrapartum eclampsia cases and the day of manifestation of neurological deficit and blindness in postpartum eclampsia cases. The prognosis and recovery details were also noted. The hospital protocol for the management of eclampsia is as follows:

Quick history is taken from the relatives and the referral letter is reviewed. Management involves initial stabilization followed by early delivery. All patients diagnosed with eclampsia are admitted to the Intensive Care Unit (ICU) of the maternity unit which is within the labour room complex. The obstetric ICU is managed by both obstetricians and anaesthetists. In order to prevent maternal injury and aspiration, the patients are nursed in the recovery position with oral suction applied and precautions are taken to prevent falling from the cot and biting of the tongue.

The airway is secured, oxygen is delivered via face mask at 4 L/minute. Continuous monitoring of the pulse, blood pressure, respiratory rate and oxygen saturation was carried out. Two intravenous lines are inserted. An indwelling catheter is inserted and a bedside test for proteinuria is done from the catheter specimen of urine. A blood sample is obtained for investigations, such as a full blood count, platelet count, coagulation profile, renal function tests, and liver function tests. Patients are monitored continuously, and invasive hemodynamic monitoring is considered only in patients with intractable cardiac failure, severe renal disease, refractory hypertension, pulmonary oedema, and oliguria. Magnesium sulphate is the drug of choice used in our hospitals for the control and prevention of seizures. A Pritchard regimen is followed for magnesium therapy. The majority of cases are referrals from other hospitals and based on the referral letters, the details of magnesium therapy prior to admission was noted. Intravenous labetalol is the commonly used antihypertensive and the aim is to keep the systolic pressure <150 mm of Hg and the diastolic pressure between 90 and 100 mm of Hg. In all cases a neurological examination was carried out by the Neuro Physician and the findings were noted. A thorough ophthalmological and fundus examination was carried out by the Ophthalmologist. Ventilatory support is given to patients who are admitted in an unconscious state when the seizures are uncontrollable and in women who have developed pulmonary oedema.

After initial resuscitation and stabilization, the mode of delivery was decided for women with intrapartum and antepartum eclampsia. Women in labour are closely monitored with the aid of a partograph and labour augmented with oxytocin if there is slow progress using an infusion pump. Those with an unfavourable cervix are offered caesarean section. If there is no contraindication to vaginal delivery, and the cervix is favourable, labour is induced by amniotomy and oxytocin infusion. The second stage of labour is shortened by vacuum or obstetrics forceps. Active management of the third stage of labour is practised to prevent postpartum haemorrhage. Patients are kept in the ICU for 48 hours after delivery /after the last fit and then shifted to the step down ward. Clinical findings are periodically reviewed for the progression or regression of neurological conditions.

Routine neuro-imaging is not carried out in all cases of eclampsia in our hospital. Only those who developed focal neurological deficit and blindness, those who are unconscious, those presenting with recurrent fits in spite of effective magnesium therapy and those with atypical presentation underwent neuroimaging within 24 hours. If required, patients are referred to other facilities for MRI studies. They are closely monitored by a team of doctors consisting of an Obstetrician, Anaesthesiologist, Neuro Physician, Nephrologist and Ophthalmologist. And after discharge, they are followed up at the respective specialty units. In those presenting with blindness, visual acuity, visual field testing and fundus examinations were carried out every 72 hours thereafter weekly until recovery. After discharge, evaluation is carried out at 6 months and one year.

Statistical Analysis

Neurological complication was considered as an outcome of interest. Those eclampsia patients with outcomes of interest were referred to as cases and those without outcomes of interest were referred to as controls. Patient's characteristics, medical and eclampsia complications were considered as explanatory variables. Descriptive analysis was carried out by frequency and proportion for categorical variables. Mean, standard deviation, median and range were also calculated for quantitative variables. Data collected were entered into the computer and an IBM SPSS version 22 was used for statistical analysis [15]. Data were analysed using logistic regression. Crude odds ratio (cOR) and 95% CIs for possible risk factors for neurological complications and blindness in women with eclampsia were calculated using univariate analysis. P value < 0.05 was considered statistically significant. Only risk factors with a P-value < 0.05 were fed into a multiple logistic regression model to obtain adjusted odds ratio (aOR) and to determine the independent contributors for neurological deficits and blindness.

RESULT

The total number of deliveries for the study period was 104,989 and 902 patients were diagnosed with eclampsia giving an institutional incidence of 0.86% and among them, 76 patients (8.4%) developed focal neurological deficits and blindness. Except for 12 patients (15.8%) who had been attending the AN clinic of the hospital regularly, 64 patients (84.2%) were referred from other facilities such as PHC, Private Nursing Homes and Corporation Hospital. 96.1% of cases had a prior history of pre-eclampsia and 3.9% had atypical presentation.

Demographic and Obstetrical Characteristics (Table 1)

In eclamptic patients with neurological complications, the mean age of presentation was 24.91 ± 5.47 years and the range was 17 to 45 years. Nearly 50% of cases were less than 24 years of age. 44 of the 76 (57.9%) women were first time pregnancies or delivered mothers. Seizures and neurological manifestations occurred in the antepartum and intrapartum period in 43 patients (56.6%) and in the postpartum period in 33 (43.4%) patients. Three patients had atypical presentation, one in the antepartum period and two in the postpartum period.

Table 1. Characteristics of eclamptic women who developed neurological complications (N = 76)

Patient's characteristics		Frequency	Percentage (%)
Age group in years	17 to 19	12	15.8
	20 to 24	26	34.2
	25 to 29	24	31.6
	30 to 34	6	7.9
	>35	8	10.5
Parity	Para 0	28	36.8
	Para 1	22	28.9
	Para 2	19	25
	Para 3	7	9.2
Timing of eclampsia	Antepartum	33	43.4
	Intrapartum	10	13.2
	Postpartum	33	43.4
Gestational age at delivery	< 28 weeks	8	10.5
	29 to 32 weeks	14	18.4
	33 to 36 weeks	36	47.4
	>37 weeks	18	23.7
Systolic BP in mm of Hg	<160	40	52.6
	161 to 180	18	23.7
	>181	18	23.7
Diastolic BP in mm of Hg	80 to 110	39	51.3
	111 to 140	30	39.5
	>140	7	9.2
Proteinuria	Nil, 1+	9	11.8
	2+, 3+, 4+	67	88.2
Associated medical conditions	Anaemia	41	53.9
	APLA	3	3.9
	GDM	3	3.9
	Cardiac disease	1	1.3
Obstetrical complications	Abruption	4	5.3
	PPH	3	3.9
Eclampsia related complications	HELLP syndrome	6	7.9
	DIVC	3	3.9
	Renal failure	4	5.3

Gestational age at delivery was < 28 weeks in 10.5% of cases, between 29 to 32 weeks in 18.4% of cases, between 33 to 36 weeks in 47.4% of cases and > 37 weeks in 23.7% of cases. On analysing the severity of the

BP, the mean systolic BP was 166.89 ± 24.95 and the range was between 120-250 mm of Hg. In 52.6% of patients, the systolic BP was <160 mm of Hg, 23,7% had BP between 161-180 mm of Hg, and the systolic BP was > 180 mm of Hg in 23.7% of cases. The mean diastolic BP was 114.83 ± 16.34 and the range was between 80-170 mm of Hg. 51.3% of patients had diastolic BP was between 80-110 mm of Hg, in 39.5% between 111 and 140 mm of Hg and in 9.2% of cases the diastolic BP was > 140 mm of Hg. Except for nine patients (11.8%), all the others 67 (88.2%) showed significant proteinuria. In 14 patients (18.4%) there was 4+ proteinuria.

Nearly 53.9% of patients suffered from anaemia. Among them, 63% of patients had moderate to severe anaemia. APLA was positive in 3.9% of patients and GDM was positive in 3 patients (3.9%). There was one case of heart disease complicating pregnancy. There were also other complications related to eclampsia with HELLP syndrome in 6 patients (7.9%), DIVC in 3 patients (3.9%) and renal failure in 4 patients (5.3%). There were four cases of abruption (5.3%) and 3 cases (3.9%) of PPH.

Neurological Manifestations in Eclamptic Patients (Table 2)

The major neurological complications noted in this study were hemiparesis/hemiplegia as seen in 57.9% of cases, followed by facial palsy in 21.1% of cases. Aphasia was present in 14.5% and ophthalmoparesis in 3.9% cases. Cortical blindness was noted in 22 patients (28.9%) and in 3 patients there was blindness due to retinal detachment. Headache was the preceding symptom in 67 patients (88%), and the other symptoms that were reported were blurring of vision, vomiting and epigastric pain. The duration of preceding symptoms was between 2 hours to 2 days and majority of patients (56.6%) had symptoms between 2-6 hours. At the initial neurological evaluation, all were at varying stages of altered sensorium, with hyper reflexes and bilateral plantar extensor. 29 (38.2%) patients were unconscious at the time of initial evaluation. 56.6% of patients had >3 seizures.

Table 2. Clinical presentation of eclamptic patients with neurological complications (N = 76)

Clinical presentation		Frequency	Percentage (%)
Neurological complications	Hemiparesis/hemiplegia	44	57.9
	Facial Palsy	16	21.1
	Aphasia	11	14.5
	Ophthalmoparesis	3	3.9
	Cortical blindness	22	28.9
	Retinal detachment	3	3.9
Preceding symptoms	Headache	36	47.4
	Vomiting	2	2.6
	Blurring	6	7.9
	Headache +Vomiting	8	10.5
	Headache+Blurring	15	19.7
	Headache+Vomiting+Blurring	7	9.2
	Epigastric pain+Vomiting	1	1.3
Duration of symptoms	<2 Hours	11	14.5
	2-6 Hours	43	56.6
	6-12 hours	16	21.1
	1 day	5	6.6
	2 days	1	1.3
Level of consciousness	Conscious	47	61.8
	Unconscious	29	38.2
Number of Seizures	<=2	33	43.4
	3-4	29	38.2
	>=5	14	18.4
Fits to admission interval (AP&IP) (43)	<=4 hours	32	74.4
	5 to 8 hours	8	18.6
	9 to 12 hours	1	2.3
	>12 hours	2	4.7
Fits to delivery interval (43)	<4 hours	3	7
	4 to 8 hours	25	58.1
	9 to 12 hours	14	32.6
	>12 hours	1	2.3
Timing of postpartum manifestation (33)	<=12 hours	9	27.3
	13 to 24 hrs	9	27.3
	2 to 4 days	9	27.3
	5 to 8 days	3	9.1
	>8 days	3	9.1

Most of the of antepartum and intrapartum eclampsia patients (74.4%) were admitted within 4 hours of seizures and 58.1% were delivered within 8 hours of admission. Among the postpartum eclampsia cases, neurological deficit manifested anywhere between 12 hours to 14 days postpartum. In 54.6% of cases neurological deficits occurred within 24 hours of delivery.

Fundus Changes (Table 3)

The ophthalmoscopic examination showed normal findings in 34.2% of cases, and 50% of cases had ≥ grade 2 retinopathy. Two patients showed evidence of papilledema and in three patients, retinal detachment was diagnosed. In the first patient diagnosed with papilledema, CT imaging showed CVT in the postpartum period and the papilledema resolved in two weeks time. The second patient was a 20 year old primigravida at 34 weeks gestation presented with 4 episodes of seizures. Her highest BP was 250/170 mm of Hg and after stabilization with antihypertensives and magnesium sulphate, emergency caesarean section was done. The CT imaging showed cerebral oedema. The patient recovered and the papilledema resolved in 14 days.

Table 3. Fundus changes in eclamptic patients with neurological complications (N = 76)

Fundus changes	Frequency	Percentage (%)
Normal	26	34.2
Grade 1 retinopathy	10	13.2
Grade 2 retinopathy	15	19.7
Grade 3 retinopathy	16	21.1
Grade 4 retinopathy	7	9.2
Papilledema	2	2.6

Neuro Imaging Findings (Table 4)

CT scan imaging was carried out in all the patients and MRI was available only in three patients. On neuroimaging, 23 patients (30.2%) were diagnosed with arterial infarcts, 10 (13.1%) were diagnosed with intracerebral haemorrhage CVT and PRES in 8 cases each (10.5%) and cerebral oedema in 14 (18.4%) cases. Neuroimaging studies were reported normal in 13 patients (17.1%).

Table 4. Showing neuro imaging findings

Finding	No.	%
Arterial infarcts	23	30.2%
Intra cerebral haemorrhage	10	13.1%
Cerebral vein thrombosis	8	10.5%
PRES	8	10.5%
Cerebral oedema	14	18.4%
Normal findings	13	17.1%

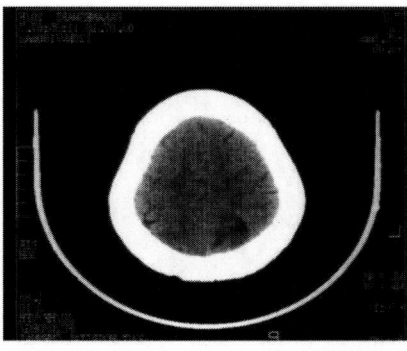

Figure 1. Plain CT axial section at the level of centrum semiovale shows a focal area of hypodensity with loss of grey white matter differentiation in left high parietal region, likely infarct.

Among the 23 patients diagnosed with arterial infarcts, 13 cases (56.5%) occurred in the antepartum period and 10 cases (43.5%) occurred in the postpartum period. Left middle cerebral artery was involved in 17 patients and posterior cerebral artery was involved in 6 patients. The CT scan imaging findings included focal loss of the normal borderline between the gray matter and white matter of brain and low attenuation in the arterial territory zones (Figure 1) and MRI imaging shows high intensity lesions (Figure 2).

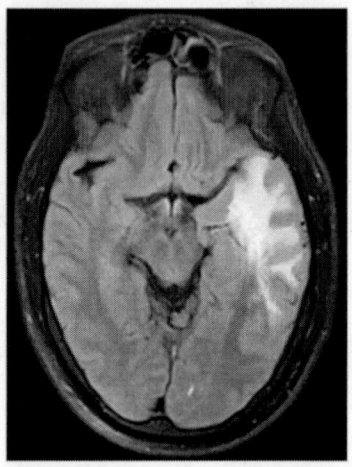

Figure 2. Axial FLAIR shows FLAIR hyperintensity with loss of grey white matter differentiation in left temporal lobe, likely infarct.

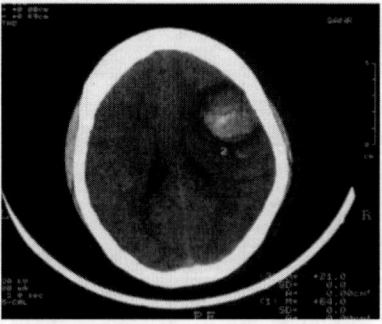

Figure 3. Plain CT axial section at the level of bilateral corona radiata shows intraparenchmal haemorrhage with mild perilesional edema in left fronto-parietal region causing mass effect in the form of effacement of adjacent cortical sulci.

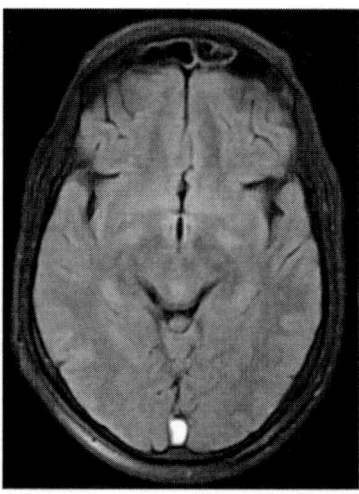

Figure 4. Axial FLAIR image shows hyperintensity, suggestive of loss of flow void in superior sagittal sinus in the posterior intercerbral fissure, likely thrombosis.

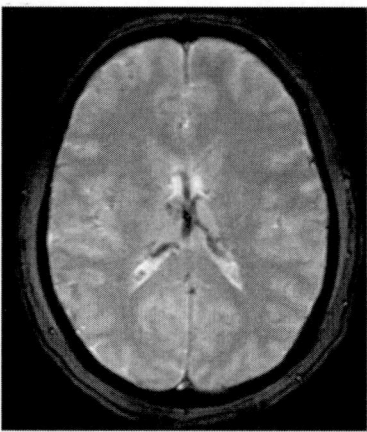

Figure 5. GRE Axial image at the level of bilateral lateral ventricles showing a linear serpiginous blooming lesion within the left lateral ventricle – suggestive of thrombosed cortical vein.

Intracerebral haemorrhage was diagnosed in 10 patients, 4 in the antepartum period and 6 in the postpartum period. CT imaging showed hyperintense lesion (Figure 3).

Eight patients were diagnosed with CVT, 2 in the antepartum period and six in the postpartum period. CT was the imaging modality in all patients and in two patients MRI was also done. Among the two cases which occurred in the antepartum period, APLA was positive in one case. The CT imaging features were infarctions in a non-arterial distribution in the white matter. In one patient who had MRI, Axial FLAIR showed thrombus in superior sagittal sinus (Figure 4).

In another patient GRE Axial image showed thrombosed cortical vein and areas of haemorrhage (Figure 5).

Eight patients were diagnosed with PRES, five in the antenatal period and three in the postpartum period. At CT imaging, the diagnosis of PRES was made by the presence of focal regions of symmetrical oedema predominantly in the parietal and occipital lobes. 14 patients (18.4%) were diagnosed with cerebral oedema and in 13 patients (17.1%) the findings were reported normal. In these patients only CT scan imaging was available.

Neurological Sequelae in Relation to Pathology in the Antenatal Period (Figure 6)

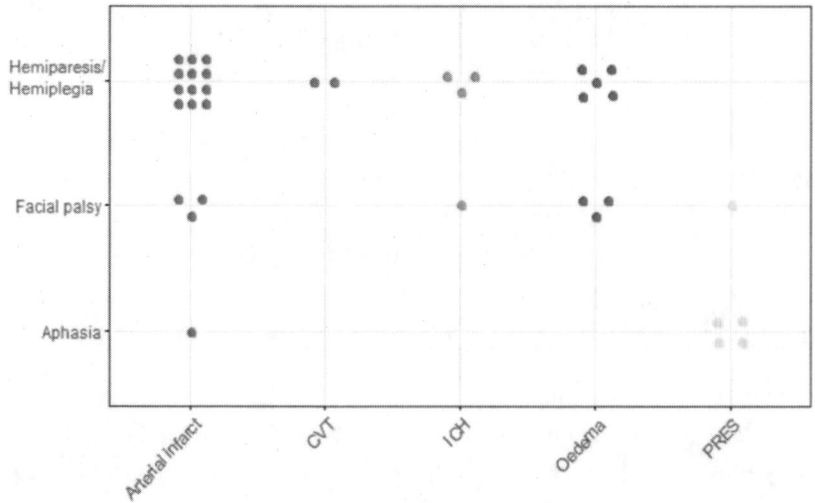

Figure 6. Neurological sequelae in relation to pathology in the antenatal period.

In the antenatal period, arterial infarcts, ICH, CVT and cerebral oedema predominantly manifested as hemiparesis/hemiplegia with or without facial palsy. There were also isolated cases of facial palsy and aphasia. PRES manifested as aphasia in 4 cases and facial palsy in 1 case. There were 13 cases of cortical blindness which manifested in the antepartum and intrapartum period and the neuroimaging findings were PRES, cerebral oedema, arterial infarcts and normal findings.

Day of Manifestation of Neurological Complications in the Postpartum Period (Figure 7)

57.6% of neurological complications which occurred in the postpartum period manifested on day 1 and 21.2% of cases manifested on day 2. All neurological manifestations were noted within 2 weeks of delivery. The day of manifestation in relation to pathology showed that neurological manifestations due to arterial infarcts, ICH, oedema and PRES manifested within 48 hours of delivery. Whereas CVT manifestations were seen up to 14 days postpartum.

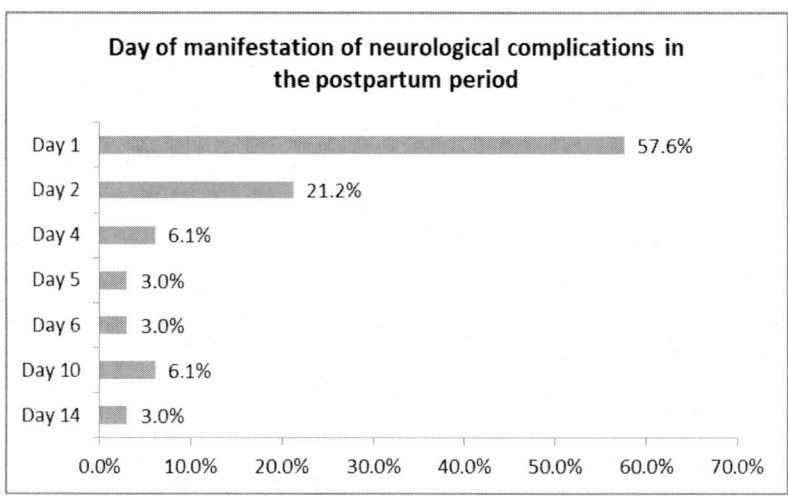

Figure 7. Day of manifestation of neurological complications in postpartum period.

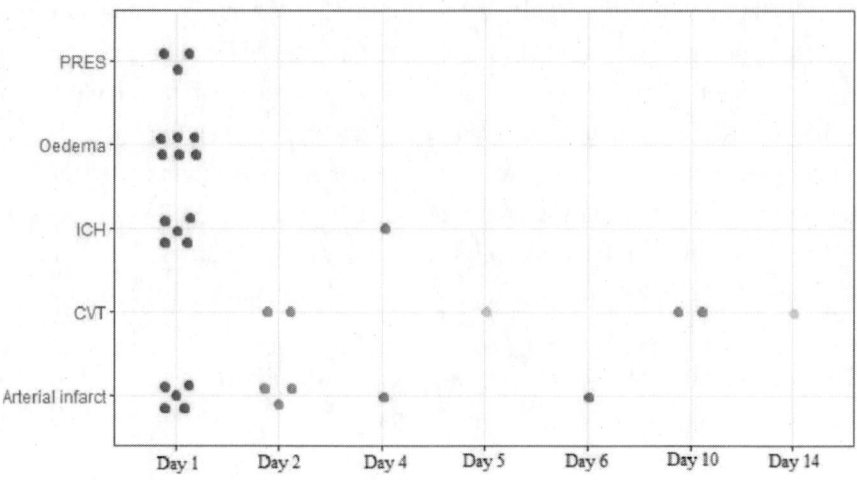

Figure 8. Day of manifestation in relation to pathology during postpartum period.

The fits to delivery interval was also assessed in patients with antepartum and intrapartum eclampsia. The mean fit to delivery interval for patients with antepartum eclampsia was 6.82 hours (SD 2.65) and was 4.80 hours (SD 1.48) for patients with intrapartum eclampsia. Among the 43 cases who were admitted with antepartum and intrapartum eclampsia, 18 (41.8%) patients were delivered by the vaginal route and 25 (58.1%) were delivered by caesarean section.

Risk Factor Analysis (Table 5)

In order to identify risk factors which can predict the occurrence of neurological complications in eclampsia, univariate analysis was carried out and it showed that age group, timing of eclampsia, diastolic blood pressure (DBP), systolic blood pressure (SBP), parity, gravidity, number of seizures, level of consciousness, fundus changes, preceding symptoms and HELLP were significant predictors of neurological complications in eclampsia patients.

Table 5. Univariate analysis for the determinants of neurological complications in eclampsia patients

Characteristics		Cases (%)	Control (%)	Univariate model cOR (95% CI)	P-value
Age group	17 to 19 (Reference)	12(15.8)	18(9.2)	1.00	
	20 to 24	26(34.2)	105(53.8)	0.37(0.16-0.87)	0.022*
	25 to 29	24(31.6)	46(23.6)	0.78(0.32-1.89)	0.586
	30 to 34	6(7.9)	17(8.7)	0.53(0.16-1.73)	0.292
	>=35	8(10.5)	9(4.6)	1.33(0.40-4.43)	0.639
Parity	0 (Reference)	28(36.8)	119(61)	1.00	
	1	22(28.9)	55(28.2)	1.70(0.89-3.23)	0.106
	2 to 3	26(34.2)	21(10.8)	5.26(2.59-10.67)	0.000*
Gestational age	>=37 weeks (Reference)	18(23.7)	40(20.5)	1.00	
	33 to 36 weeks	36(47.4)	82(42.1)	0.98(0.49-1.93)	0.943
	29 to 32 weeks	14(18.4)	38(19.5)	0.82(0.36-1.87)	0.636
	<=28 weeks	8(10.5)	35(17.9)	0.51(0.20-1.31)	0.162
Timing of eclampsia	Antepartum (Reference)	33(43.4)	136(69.7)	1.00	
	Intrapartum	10(13.2)	14(7.2)	2.94(1.20-7.21)	0.018*
	Postpartum	33(43.4)	45(23.1)	3.02(1.68-5.44)	0.000*
SBP	<=160 (Reference)	40(52.6)	128(65.6)	1.00	
	>160	36(47.4)	67(34.4)	1.72(1.00-2.95)	0.049*
DBP	80 to 110 (Reference)	39(51.3)	140(71.8)	1.00	
	>110	37(48.7)	55(28.2)	2.41(1.40-4.17)	0.002*
Number of Seizures	<=2 (Reference)	33(43.4)	115(59)	1.00	
	3 to 4	29(38.2)	69(35.4)	1.46(0.82-2.62)	0.198
	>=5	14(18.4)	11(5.6)	4.44(1.84-10.69)	0.001*
Coma	Conscious (Reference)	47(61.8)	184(94.4)	1.00	
	Unconscious	29(38.2)	11(5.6)	10.32(4.81-22.17)	0.000*
Fundus changes	Normal (Reference)	26(34.2)	109(55.9)	1.00	
	GR I	10(13.2)	39(20)	1.07(0.48-2.43)	0.862
	GR II	15(19.7)	25(12.8)	2.52(1.16-5.43)	0.019
	GR III	16(21.1)	19(9.7)	3.53(1.60-7.78)	0.002
	GR IV	7(9.2)	1(0.5)	29.35(3.46-249.05)	0.002
	Papilloedema	2(2.6)	2(1.0)	4.19(0.56-31.17)	0.161
Preceding symptoms	Headache (Reference)	36(47.4)	110(56.4)	1.00	
	Blurring	6(7.9)	10(5.1)	1.83(0.62-5.40)	0.271
	Vomiting	2(2.6)	4(2.1)	1.53(0.27-8.69)	0.633

Table 5. (Continued)

Characteristics		Cases (%)	Control (%)	Univariate model cOR (95% CI)	P-value
	E+V	1(1.3)	3(1.5)	1.02(0.10-10.10)	0.987
	H+B	15(19.7)	15(7.7)	3.06(1.36-6.86)	0.007*
	H+E+V	1(1.3)	2(1.0)	1.53(0.13-17.35)	0.732
	H+V	8(10.5)	7(3.6)	3.49(1.18-10.30)	0.023*
	H+V+B	7(9.2)	9(4.6)	2.38(0.83-6.84)	0.108
	Breathlessness	0(0.0)	5(2.6)	-	0.993
	Oliguria	0(0.0)	4(2.1)	-	0.993
	H+oliguria	0(0.0)	5(2.5)	-	0.994
	H+E	0(0.0)	3(1.5)	-	0.994
	None	0(0.0)	18(9.2)	-	0.986
Anaemia	No (Reference)	35(46.1)	82(42.1)	1.00	
	Mild	15(19.7)	29(14.9)	1.21(0.58-2.54)	0.610
	Moderate	24(31.6)	74(37.9)	0.76(0.41-1.39)	0.375
	Severe	2(2.6)	10(5.1)	0.47(0.10-2.25)	0.344
DIVC	No (Reference)	73(96.1)	194(99.5)	1.00	
	Yes	3(3.9)	1(0.5)	7.97(0.82-77.88)	0.074
HELLP	No (Reference)	70(92.1)	191(97.9)	1.00	
	Yes	6(7.9)	4(2.1)	4.09(1.12-14.93)	0.033*
Renal failure	No (Reference)	72(94.7)	191(97.9)	1.00	
	Yes	4(5.3)	4(2.1)	2.65(0.65-10.89)	0.176
Pulmonary oedema	No (Reference)	76(100.0)	193(99.0)	1.00	
	Yes	0(0.0)	2(1.0)	-	0.989
PPH	No (Reference)	73(96.1)	192(98.5)	1.00	
	Yes	3(3.9)	3(1.5)	2.63(0.52-13.33)	0.243
Abruption	No (Reference)	72(94.7)	189(96.9)	1.00	
	Yes	4(5.3)	6(3.1)	1.75(0.48-6.38)	0.397
Fits to Admission interval (AP and IP)	<=4 hours (Reference)	32(74.4)	106(70.7)	1.00	
	5 to 8 hours	8(18.6)	41(27.3)	0.65(0.28-1.52)	0.317
	9 to 12 hours	1(2.3)	2(1.3)	1.66(0.15-18.87)	0.684
	>12 hours	2(4.7)	1(0.7)	6.63(0.58-75.46)	0.128
Timing of postpartum manifestation	<=12 hours (Reference)	9(27.3)	24(53.3)	1.00	
	13 to 24 hrs	9(27.3)	10(22.2)	2.40(0.74-7.83)	0.147
	2 to 4 days	9(27.3)	7(15.6)	3.43(0.98-11.97)	0.053
	5 to 8 days	3(9.1)	3(6.7)	2.67(0.45-15.72)	0.279
	>8 days	3(9.1)	1(2.2)	8.00(0.73-87.25)	0.088

Characteristics		Cases (%)	Control (%)	Univariate model	
				cOR (95% CI)	P-value
Fits to delivery interval (Only for AP and IP)	<4 hours (Reference)	3(7.0)	16(10.9)	1.00	
	4 to 7 hours	25(58.1)	96(65.3)	1.39(0.38-5.14)	0.543
	8 to 12 hours	14(32.6)	31(21.1)	2.41(0.60-9.62)	0.214
	>12 hours	1(2.3)	4(2.7)	1.33(0.11-16.48)	0.823

Note: * Statistically significant (p < 0.05); cOR: Crude Odds Ratio.
E+V - Epigastric pain and vomiting.
H+B - Headache and blurring.
H+E+V - Headache+epigastric pain and vomiting.

Patients from age group 20 to 24 were 63% (cOR 0.37, 95% CI 0.16-0.87) less likely to develop neurological complication as compared to patients from age group 17 to 19. Patients with intrapartum eclampsia and postpartum eclampsia were 2.94 times (cOR 2.94, 95% CI 1.20-7.21) and 3.02 times (cOR 3.02, 95% CI 1.68-5.44) respectively, more likely to develop neurological complications as compared to patients with antepartum eclampsia. Patients with SBP greater than 160 mmHg were 1.72 times (cOR 1.72, 95% CI 1.00-2.95) more likely to develop neurological complications as compared to patients with SBP <=160 mmHg. Patients with DBP greater than 110 mmHg were 2.41 times (cOR 2.41, 95% CI 1.40-4.17) more likely to develop neurological complications as compared to patients with DBP 80-110 mmHg. As compared to patients with primigravida, patients with multigravida were 3.03 times (cOR 3.84, 95% CI 2.17-6.82) more likely to develop neurological complications. Patients with para 2 to 3 were 5.26 times (cOR 5.26, 95% CI 2.59-10.67) more likely to develop neurological complications as compared to nulliparous patients. Patients with number of seizures >=5 were 4.44 times (cOR 4.44, 95% CI 1.84-10.69) more likely to develop neurological complications as compared to patients with number of seizures <=2. As compared to conscious patients, unconscious patients were 10.32 times (cOR 10.32, 95% CI 4.81-22.17) more likely to develop neurological complications. Patients with grade 2 retinopathy, grade 3 retinopathy and grade 4 retinopathy were 2.52 times(cOR 2.52 95% CI 1.16-5.43), 3.53 times (cOR 3.53 95% CI 1.60-7.78) and 29.35 times (cOR 29.35 95% CI

3.46-249.05) respectively, more likely to develop neurological complications as compared to normal patients. The high odds ratio in grade 4 retinopathy is due to just 1 patient in the control group. As compared to patients with the preceding symptom headache, patients with headache and blurring (H+B) and headache and vomiting (H+V) were 3.06 times (cOR 3.06 95% CI 1.36-6.86) and 3.49 times (cOR 3.49, 95% CI 1.18-10.30) respectively, more likely to develop neurological complications. Patients with HELLP syndrome were 4.09 times (cOR 4.09 95% CI 1.12-14.93) more likely to develop neurological complications as compared to patients without HELLP syndrome.

Univariate analysis showed that patients with postpartum eclampsia who gave birth by vaginal delivery were 4.30 times (cOR 4.30 95% CI 1.49-12.43) more likely to develop neurological complication as compared to patients with postpartum eclampsia who gave birth by caesarean section (Table 6).

Table 6. Mode of delivery in patients with postpartum eclampsia

Mode of delivery	Group		cOR (95% CI)	P-value
	Cases (Complication)	Controls (No complication)		
Caesarean section (Reference)	6 (18.2)	22 (48.9)	4.30(1.49-12.43)	0.007*
Vaginal delivery	27 (81.8)	23 (51.1)		

Independent Risk Factor Analysis (Table 7)

In order to identify the independent risk factors for the occurrence of neurological complications in eclampsia, multivariate logistic regression analysis was done. Table 7 shows the results from binary logistic regression analysis for neurological complications in eclampsia patients. Some of the variables were re-categorized in the logistic regression due to zero/low frequency in certain categories. Parity was not included in the multivariate model due to multicollinearity problems. Both univariate and multivariate models showed that age group, timing of eclampsia, diastolic blood pressure (DBP) and gravidity were significant predictors of neurological complications in eclampsia patients.

Table 7. Multivariate analysis for the determinants of neurological complications in eclampsia patients

Characteristics		Univariate model		Multivariate model	
		cOR (95% CI)	P-value	aOR (95% CI)	P-value
Age group	17 to 19 (Reference)	1.00		1.00	
	20 to 24	0.37(0.16-0.87)	0.022*	0.16(0.06-0.46)	0.001*
	25 to 29	0.78(0.32-1.89)	0.586	0.29(0.09-0.87)	0.027*
	30 to 34	0.53(0.16-1.73)	0.292	0.19(0.05-0.81)	0.025*
	>=35	1.33(0.40-4.43)	0.639	0.47(0.11-2.03)	0.309
Timing of eclampsia	Antepartum (Reference)	1.00		1.00	
	Intrapartum	2.94(1.20-7.21)	0.018*	3.74(1.31-10.70)	0.014*
	Postpartum	3.02(1.68-5.44)	0.000*	3.18(1.36-7.45)	0.008*
SBP	<=160 (Reference)	1.00		1.00	
	>160	1.72(1.00-2.95)	0.049*	1.25(0.61-2.57)	0.544
DBP	80 to 110 (Reference)	1.00		1.00	
	>110	2.41(1.40-4.17)	0.002*	2.82(1.34-5.91)	0.006*
Gravidity	1 (Reference)	1.00		1.00	
	2 or more	3.84(2.17-6.82)	0.000*	3.03(1.27-7.23)	0.012*
Parity	0 Reference)	1.00			
	1	1.70(0.89-3.23)	0.106		
	2 to 3	5.26(2.59-10.67)	0.000*		

From the multivariate model, patients from age groups 20 to 24, 25 to 29 and 30 to 34 were 84% (aOR 0.16, 95% CI 0.06-0.46), 71% (aOR 0.29, 95% CI 0.09-0.87) and 81% (aOR 0.19, 95% CI 0.05-0.81) respectively, less likely to develop neurological complication as compared to patients from age group 17 to 19. Patients with intrapartum eclampsia and postpartum eclampsia were 3.74 times (aOR 3.74, 95% CI 1.31-10.70) and 3.18 times (aOR 3.18, 95% CI 1.96-7.45) respectively, more likely to develop neurological complications as compared to patients with antepartum eclampsia in the adjusted analysis. Patients with DBP greater than 110 were 2.82 times (aOR 2.82, 95% CI 1.34-5.91) more likely to develop neurological complications as compared to patients with DBP 80-110. As compared to patients with primigravida, patients with multigravida were 3.03 times (aOR 3.03, 95% CI 1.27-7.23) more likely to develop neurological complications.

In order to identify the risk factors for the occurrence of arterial infarcts, ICH and CVT leading to neurological deficit in eclampsia, binary logistic regression was done.

Determinants of Arterial Infarcts in Eclampsia Patients (Table 8)

Assessing the risk factors for arterial infarcts in eclampsia, in the univariate model, none of the predictors were found to be significant (p>0.05). However, diastolic blood pressure (DBP) was found significant in the multivariate model. Patients with DBP greater than 110 were 3.29 times (aOR 3.29, 95% CI 1.14-9.52) more likely to develop arterial infarcts as compared to patients with DBP 80-110.

Table 8. Determinants of Arterial infarcts in eclampsia patients

Characteristics		Arterial infarcts		Univariate model		Multivariate model	
		Yes (%)	No (%)	cOR (95% CI)	P-value	aOR (95% CI)	P-value
Timing of eclampsia	AP (Reference)	12(52.2)	157(63.3)	1.00		1.00	
	PP	11(47.8)	67(27)	2.15(0.90-5.11)	0.084	2.33(0.93-5.83)	0.071
SBP	<=160 (Reference)	15(65.2)	153(61.7)	1.00		1.00	
	>160	8(34.8)	95(38.3)	0.86(0.35-2.10)	0.739	0.48(0.16-1.45)	0.194
DBP	80 to 110 (Reference)	12(52.2)	167(67.3)	1.00		1.00	
	>110	11(47.8)	81(32.7)	1.89(0.80-4.47)	0.147	3.29(1.14-9.52)	0.028*
Anaemia	No (Reference)	6(26.1)	111(44.8)	1.00		1.00	
	Yes	17(73.9)	137(55.2)	2.30(0.88-6.02)	0.091	2.37(0.88-6.41)	0.088

Note: * Statistically significant (p < 0.05); cOR: Crude Odds Ratio; aOR: Adjusted Odds Ratio.

Determinants of ICH in Eclampsia Patients (Table 9)

Binary logistic regression was done to assess the risk factors for ICH in eclampsia patients. In both univariate and multivariate models, the timing of eclampsia was found to be a significant predictor of ICH. SBP was also found to be significant in the multivariate model. From the multivariate model, patients with postpartum eclampsia were 6.44 times (aOR 6.44, 95% CI 1.52-27.32) more likely to develop ICH as compared to patients with antepartum eclampsia. As compared to patients with SBP less than equal to 160, patients with SBP greater than 160 were 5.75 times (aOR 5.75, 95% CI 1.31-25.19) more likely to develop ICH in the adjusted analysis.

Determinants of CVT in Eclampsia Patients (Table 10)

By both univariate and multivariate models, the timing of eclampsia was found to be a significant predictor of CVT. Patients with postpartum eclampsia were 9.59 times (aOR 9.59, 95% CI 2.00-46.08) more likely to develop CVT as compared to patients with antepartum eclampsia in the adjusted analysis.

Table 9. Determinants of ICH in eclampsia patients

Characteristics		Univariate model		Multivariate model	
		cOR (95% CI)	P-value	aOR (95% CI)	P-value
Timing of eclampsia	AP (Reference)	1.00		1.00	
	PP	5.46(1.37-21.70)	0.016*	6.44(1.52-27.32)	0.012*
SBP	<=160 (Reference)	1.00		1.00	
	>160	2.99(0.85-10.48)	0.087	5.75(1.31-25.19)	0.020*
DBP	80 to 110 (Reference)	1.00		1.00	
	>110	1.12(0.32-3.92)	0.863	0.77(0.18-3.34)	0.726
Anaemia	No (Reference)	1.00		1.00	
	Yes	2.08(0.54-8.03)	0.287	2.27(0.55-9.31)	0.256

Note: * Statistically significant (p < 0.05); cOR: Crude Odds Ratio; aOR: Adjusted Odds Ratio.

Table 10. Determinants of CVT in eclampsia patients

Characteristics		Univariate model		Multivariate model	
		cOR (95% CI)	P-value	aOR (95% CI)	P-value
Timing of eclampsia	Antepartum (Reference)	1.00		1.00	
	Postpartum	10.89(2.29-51.71)	0.003*	9.59(2.00-46.08)	0.005*
SBP	<=160 (Reference)	1.00		1.00	
	>160	0.60(0.16-2.31)	0.458	1.29(0.29-5.73)	0.742
DBP	80 to 110 (Reference)	1.00		1.00	
	>110	0.19(0.02-1.47)	0.111	0.220.02-2.04)	0.182
Anaemia	No (Reference)	1.00		1.00	
	Yes	1.35(0.38-4.71)	0.643	1.10(0.30-4.07)	0.888

Note: * Statistically significant (p < 0.05); cOR: Crude Odds Ratio; aOR: Adjusted Odds Ratio.

Visual Complications in Eclampsia

The most common ocular complaint in pre-eclampsia/eclampsia is blurred vision which was seen in 36.8% of our patients. The major ocular complication associated with eclampsia in our study was blindness due to serous retinal detachments in 3 patients and cortical blindness in 22 (2.4%) patients. Blindness was the only manifestation in 16 of the 22 cases and in 6 cases there were also other neurological deficits such as hemiparesis, hemiplegia and aphasia. Blindness manifested in the antenatal period in 6 patients (27.2%), in the intrapartum period in 7 (31.8%) and in the postpartum period in 9 cases (40.9%). At the time of manifestation of blindness, seven patients were in active labour and all were delivered by the vaginal route. Six patients with antenatal manifestation were delivered by caesarean section. All patients were delivered within 4-8 hours of diagnosing blindness. Nine patients developed blindness in the postpartum period. Blindness was preceded by intense headache in 10 cases (45.5%) and the duration of preceding symptoms was 2-6 hours in 54.5% of cases. There were associated medical complications such as GDM in two patients and moderate to severe anaemia in eight patients, HELLP syndrome in one patient, renal failure and post partum haemorrhage also in one patient.

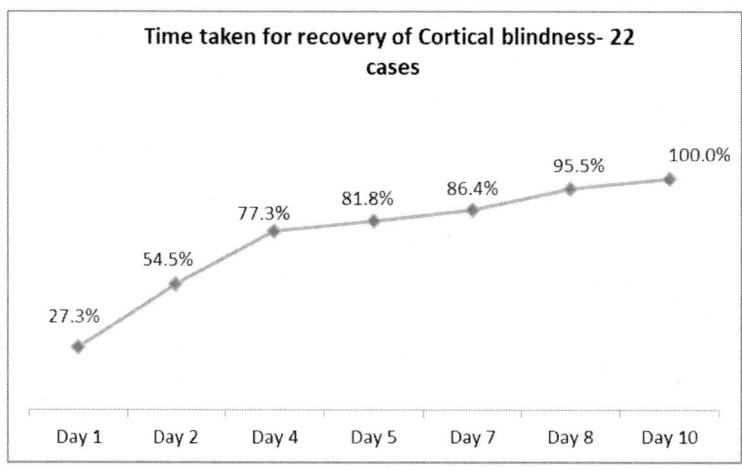

Figure 9. Time taken for recovery of cortical blindness.

Neuroimaging findings associated with cortical blindness were cerebral oedema in 10 cases, PRES in 1 case and arterial infarcts in 3 cases and 8 cases were reported normal. The duration of blindness ranged from 12 hours to 10 days. In all cases, there was a perception of bright light within 24 hours. Complete recovery was noted in as early as 12 hours. In 27.3% of cortical blindness patients, the vision recovered within 1 day. Though there was transient recovery of vision, complete recovery of vision was seen in all 22 patients with cortical blindness within 10 days (Fig 9). Visual acuity, visual field testing and fundus examinations were carried out every 72 hours. At two weeks follow up, the visual acuity, papillary reflexes and fundus examination were normal. After discharge, the 6 month and one year evaluations also remained normal.

Retinal Detachment

In three patients retinal detachment was diagnosed, and their systolic and diastolic BP were very high prior to the manifestation of blindness. In all the three patients, retinal detachment manifested in the postpartum period. All of them presented with intense headaches 2-6 hours prior to the blindness. The first patient developed continuous fits 12 hours after vaginal delivery, the systolic BP was 230 mm of Hg and the diastolic BP was 150 mm of Hg, and there was hemiplegia. The neuro imaging showed ICH and the patient could not be saved. The other two patients also had high systolic BP of 180 and 200 and the diastolic BP of 120 mm of Hg. In these two patients, the CT scan imaging showed cerebral oedema. Transient recovery of vision was noted in 2 days and complete recovery of vision occurred in 4 and 9 days.

Prognosis

The recovery time of patients who developed neurological complications was also assessed. The mean recovery time for aphasia was 3.13 weeks, hemiparesis 5.78 weeks, facial palsy 6.05 weeks, ophthamoparesis 9.05 weeks, cortical blindness 6.09 days and retinal detachment 6.5 days. 45.5% of the aphasia patients recovered within 1 week. It took 12 weeks for the recovery of speech in all 100% of cases (Figure 10).

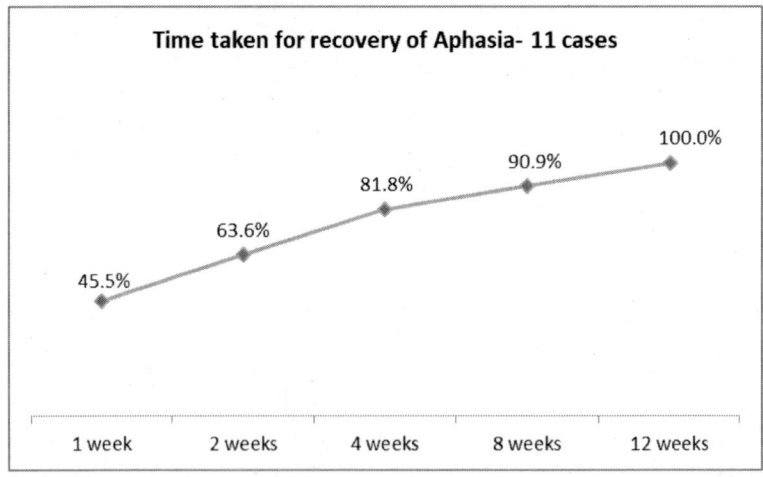

Figure 10. Time taken for recovery of aphasia.

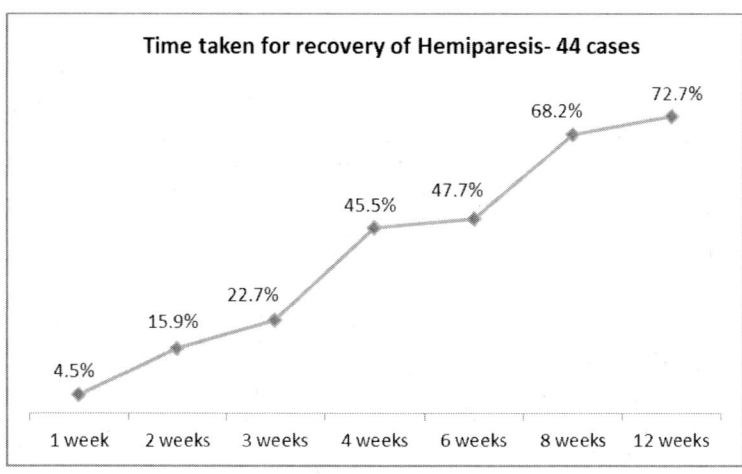

Figure 11. Time taken for recovery of hemiparesis/hemiplegia.

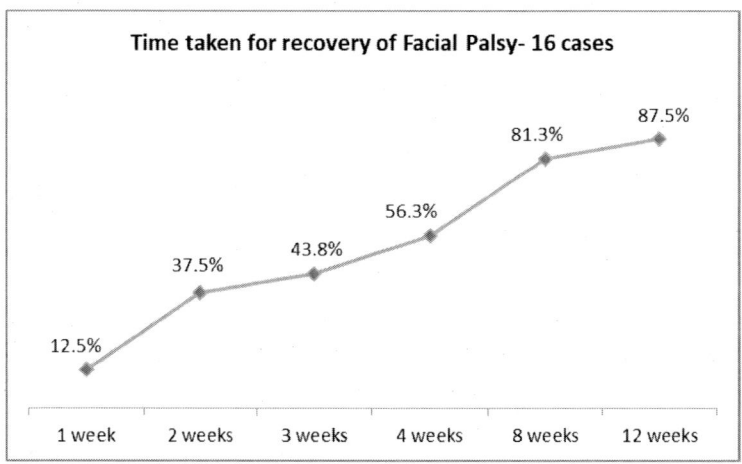

Figure 12. Time taken for recovery of facial palsy.

Only 72.7% of hemiparesis patients recovered within 12 weeks. 22.7% (10 cases) died, and 4.6% (2 case) had residual lesion at 3 months (Figure 11). Only 87.5% of facial palsy patients recovered within 12 weeks. 6.3% (1 case) died and 6.3% (1 case) had residual lesion at 3 months (Figure 12).

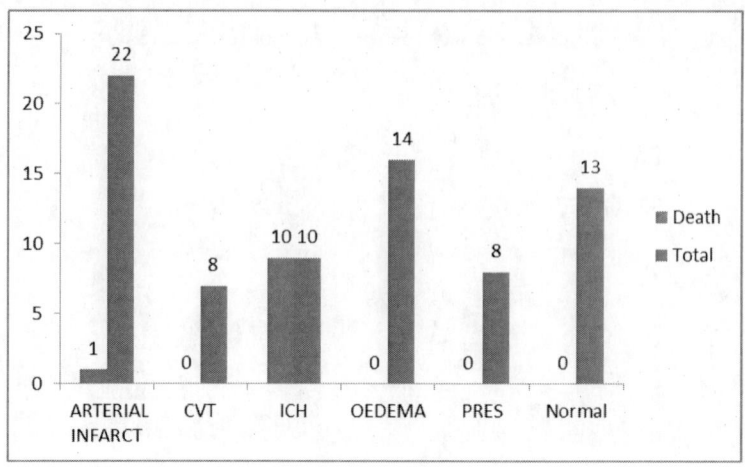

Figure 13. Death according to aetiology.

There were 11 deaths among patients with eclampsia who developed neurological complications. Among those with ICH there was 100% of death, whereas among those with arterial infarcts there was one death out of 23 cases. All patients who showed CVT, PRES and cerebral oedema recovered (Figure 13).

DISCUSSION

Pre-eclampsia and eclampsia cause significant maternal and perinatal morbidity and mortality worldwide. Preeclampsia is classified as one of the hypertensive disorders of pregnancy. It is generally defined as new onset hypertension with proteinuria during pregnancy. Preeclampsia can superimpose on pre pregnancy hypertension with worsening blood pressure and proteinuria. Eclampsia is defined as tonic-clonic seizures in a pregnant or recently delivered woman not attributable to other causes than preeclampsia or gestational hypertension, and complicates about 1 to 2% of all cases of severe preeclampsia [16]. It is a multi-system disorder secondary to generalised vasospasm and endothelial damage. Eclampsia related complications which lead to significant maternal morbidity and mortality are cerebro vascular accidents (CVA), pulmonary oedema, renal failure, HELLP (haemolysis, elevated liver enzyme, and low platelet count) syndrome, DIC (Disseminated Intravascular Coagulation) and hepatic failure [7]. It is estimated that the prevalence of pre-eclampsia globally is 4.6% (95% CI 2.7%–8.2%) [17]. There is a wide variation in the incidence of pre-eclampsia/eclampsia worldwide. In our study, the incidence of pre-eclampsia during the study period was 11.3% and that of eclampsia was 0.86%. The average annual incidence rate of eclampsia in Europe and the US vary between 0.3 and 0.6/1000 [18, 19. 20]. The prevalence of eclampsia reported by Abalos et al. globally was 0.3% [21]. The National Eclampsia Registry (NER) of India (FOGSI -ICOG) has shown that the incidence of preeclampsia is 10.3% (NER 2013) and that of eclampsia is 1.9% [22]. Compared to our national statistics, the incidence of eclampsia in our institution in this study was lower at 0.86%.

During the study period there were 906 eclampsia cases, and 76 of them (8.4%) developed focal neurological deficits and blindness. As pre-eclampsia and eclampsia are diseases of young women, neurological complications were also seen more commonly in young women; nearly 50% were less than 25 years of age and 57.9% women were first time pregnant or delivered mothers. Similar to our study, other authors have also shown that the neurological complications in eclampsia occurred more commonly in primigravid women compared to multigravid women [23, 24]. However, on logistic regression analysis compared to the primigravidae, multigravida were 3.03 times (aOR 3.03, 95% CI 1.27-7.23) more likely to develop neurological complications. There are reports to show that not all cases of eclampsia are preceded by severe pre-eclampsia [25, 26]. We had three patients who had atypical presentation and were not preceded by typical criteria for pre-eclampsia and their BP was <140/90 mm of Hg. It has been suggested that the change in blood pressure necessary to promote hyper perfusion and hydrostatic brain oedema is considerably lower in pregnancy and reports have also shown that eclampsia can occur at blood pressures that are considerably lower than those reported for hypertensive encephalopathy [27]. Seizures and neurological manifestations occurred in the antepartum and intrapartum period in 43 patients (56.6%) and in the postpartum period in 33 (43.4%) patients. Study by Martin et al. showed that the majority (57%) of strokes occurred postpartum [28].

In this study, the majority of patients had very high systolic and diastolic blood pressure prior to the onset of seizures and neurological manifestations. The mean systolic BP was 166.89 ± 24.95 and was >180 mm of Hg in 23.7% of cases. The mean diastolic BP was 114.83 ± 16.34 and in 9.2% of cases the diastolic BP was >140 mm of Hg prior to convulsion. In the study by Martin et al. the systolic pressure was 160 mm Hg or greater in 95.8% of cases and the diastolic pressure of >110 mm Hg was seen only in 12.5% of cases [28]. In our study the systolic pressure was >160 mm Hg only in 47.4% of cases and the diastolic pressure was >110 mm Hg in 48.7% of cases. There are data to suggest that the degree of hypertension is only relatively important and it is the rapidity of changes that may be of primary importance as well as the patient's customary blood pressure prior the development of hypertension [29]. There was significant proteinuria in >88% of cases indicating the severity of the condition. In India, anaemia is a very common medical problem affecting pregnant women and was seen in nearly 53.9% of patients in association with eclampsia. APLA testing is not routinely carried out in our hospital, however 3 patients had a prior diagnosis of APLA and one of these patients manifested as CVT in the antenatal period. GDM was positive in 3 patients (3.9%) and two of them manifested with cortical blindness. In the third patient, the pre-seizure BP was 230/150 mm of Hg, manifested with hemiplegia and retinal detachment and the CT imaging showed ICH. Studies have shown that GDM is associated with abnormal cerebral blood flow regulation and the rise in glucose concentration dilates cerebral arteries by an increased release of nitric oxide from the endothelium. This mechanism may counter the neurogenic and myogenic vessel tone and thereby weakening the blood-brain barrier predisposing to neurological manifestations. Leszek et al. have reported cortical blindness occurring in patients with pre-eclampsia and GDM [30]. There were also other complications related to eclampsia with HELLP syndrome in 6 patients (7.9%), DIVC in 3 patients (3.9%) and renal failure in 4 patients (5.3%). There were four cases of abruption (5.3%) and 3 cases (3.9%) of PPH. As 84.2% of patients were referred from other facilities there was a delay in initiating effective antihypertensive and anti convulsant therapy in most of the patients. However, most of the antepartum and intrapartum eclampsia patients (74.4%) were admitted within 4 hours of seizures and 58.1% were delivered within 8 hours of admission.

Various fundus changes reported in patients with pre-eclampsia /eclampsia include spasm and focal/generalized narrowing of retinal arterioles, haemorrhages, exudates, focal retinal oedema, serous retinal detachment and papilledema [31]. More than 50% of our patients showed narrowing of retinal arterioles, haemorrhages and exudates. Haemorrhages and exudates usually take 6- 8 weeks to resolve following control of blood pressure. In two patients with CVT and cerebral oedema, papilledema was diagnosed. In both cases, papilledema resolved in two weeks following control of hypertension, convulsions and delivery. Permanent loss of vision can occur due to optic atrophy secondary to papilledema. The presence of papilledema on fundoscopy is an indication for neuroimaging studies and urgent intervention. The severity of retinopathy has prognostic value and would indicate the need for terminating the pregnancy [31]. In this study, the causes of neurological deficits and blindness were found to be arterial infarcts in 30.2% of cases, intracerebral haemorrhage in 13.1% of cases, cerebral vein thrombosis in 10.5% of cases, PRES in 10.5% of cases and cerebral oedema in 18.4% of cases. In the antenatal period, arterial infarcts, ICH, CVT and cerebral oedema predominantly manifested as hemiparesis/hemiplegia with or without facial palsy. PRES predominantly manifested as aphasia, facial palsy and cortical blindness. In the postpartum period, ICH and arterial infarcts manifested early and were clustered within 6 days of delivery, whereas CVT was mostly clustered around the first and second week after delivery. A study by Srinivasan showed that CVT occurs mostly in the second week of puerperium and can be delayed for 3- 4 weeks after delivery [32].

Risk factor analysis on the univariate model showed that, age group, timing of eclampsia, diastolic blood pressure (DBP), systolic blood pressure (SBP), parity, gravidity, number of seizures, level of consciousness, fundus changes, preceding symptoms and HELLP were significant predictors of neurological complications in eclampsia patients. Independent risk factors for the occurrence of neurological complications in eclampsia was assessed using multivariate logistic regression analysis and it was found that intrapartum and postpartum eclampsia, diastolic blood pressure, multiparity and age were significant independent risk factors for the occurrence of neurological complications in eclampsia. Patients with intrapartum eclampsia and postpartum eclampsia were 3.74 times (aOR 3.74, 95% CI 1.31-10.70) and 3.18 times (aOR 3.18, 95% CI 1.96-7.45) respectively, more likely to develop neurological complications as compared to patients with antepartum eclampsia in the adjusted analysis. Patients with DBP greater than 110 were 2.82 times (aOR 2.82, 95% CI 1.34-5.91) more likely to develop neurological complications as compared to patients with DBP 80-110. As compared to patients with primigravida, patients with multigravida were 3.03 times (aOR 3.03, 95% CI 1.27-7.23) more likely to develop neurological complications.

In order to understand the neurological manifestations of pre-eclampsia/eclampsia, cerebral haemodynamics in normal pregnancy and in pre-eclampsia/eclampsia is discussed here:

Haemodynamic in Normal Pregnancy

The Circle of Willis at the base of the brain regionally distributes blood flow to the cerebral cortex. After exiting the Circle of Willis, the paired anterior, middle, and posterior cerebral arteries branch to form a network of arterioles and capillaries. The middle cerebral artery carries nearly 80% of the flow to the hemispheres of the brain. The cerebral blood flow is maintained at 60 and 150 mm of Hg by autoregulation. The cerebral autoregulation is maintained by myogenic and neurogenic mechanisms. The neurogenic component is controlled by sympathetic innervations which predominates in the anterior circulation. Compared to the anterior cerebral territories, the posterior circulation is sparsely innervated and there is uneven sympathetic innervations of cerebral circulation. In the presence of acute hypertension, the neurogenic response plays a major role in maintaining a constant cerebral perfusion by the autoregulatory mechanism [29].

Cerebrovascular Changes in Pre-Eclampsia/Eclampsia

Hypertension causes a breakdown in cerebral auto regulation leading to overdistension of blood vessels and extravasation of fluid into the perivascular space causing cerebral oedema. Hypertension also induces capillary damage and immune mediated endothelial cell dysfunction. The vasospasm induced by hypertension causes fibrinoid changes and necrosis in small blood vessels which rupture due to high blood pressure. Rupture of blood vessels can also occur due to sudden fall in BP while on antihypertensive therapy. The impaired coagulation system and deficiency of platelets caused by pre-eclampsia/eclampsia also predispose to intracranial bleeds. The resultant cerebral pathology includes cerebral oedema, micro-infarcts, cortical petechiae and pericapillary haemorrhages. Two theories have been proposed for alteration of cerebral blood flow in eclampsia; forced dilatation theory and vasospasm theory. During acute hypertension at pressures above the autoregulatory limit, the myogenic constriction of vascular smooth muscle is overcome by the excessive intravascular pressure, and forced dilatation of cerebral vessels occurs decreasing the effect of myogenic mechanism, allowing local hyper perfusion, leading to vasogenic and interstitial oedema. These changes are predominantly seen in the occipital lobe, which is transient and not associated with infarctions [33]. According to the vasospasm theory, cerebral over regulation occurs in response to hypertension, resulting in ischemia, cytotoxic oedema, cell damage and infarctions. The area supplied by the posterior circulation is most vulnerable to breakthrough of the blood–brain barrier and failure of autoregulatory mechanisms because of less sympathetic innervation and less ability for neurogenic response to increased blood pressure. Besides the generalized vasospasm, there is also systemic inflammatory response which is an inherent component of preeclamptic disease and progress in spite of blood pressure control [34, 35].

Pathogenesis of Cerebral Oedema

The cerebral oedema which develops in eclampsia is one of two types, namely cytogenic oedema and vasogenic oedema. The pathogenesis of cytotoxic oedema is that, in response to acute hypertension there is extreme vasospasm of the cerebral vasculature, resulting in decrease in cerebral blood flow and when it becomes extreme it results in ischemia, cytotoxic oedema and, eventually, tissue infarction. Vasogenic oedema develops when there is a sudden elevation in systemic blood pressure which may exceed the cerebrovascular autoregulatory capacity. When autoregulation fails, there are areas of passive vasodilation and vasoconstriction which eventually lead to an increase in hydrostatic pressure. This may result in hyper perfusion and extravasation of plasma and red cells resulting in vasogenic oedema. This phenomenon has been described as reversible posterior leukoencephalopathy syndrome (RPLS) also known as posterior reversible encephalopathy syndrome or PRES). In vasogenic oedema, there is progressive brain compression within the closed space of the skull, resulting in classic neurologic symptoms of headache, cortical blindness and convulsions and focal neurological deficits [36].

Causes of Neurological Deficits and Blindness in Eclampsia

The possible causes of focal neurological deficits and blindness in eclampsia may be due to various causes such as hemorrhagic and non-hemorrhagic stoke, cerebral oedema, and PRES [13]. The stroke in eclampsia may be due to arterial ischemia, venous thrombosis or intracerebral hemorrhage. Ischemic stroke is an episode of neurological dysfunction caused by focal cerebral infarction. The stroke caused by cerebral venous thrombosis is due to the thrombosis of a cerebral venous structure leading to oedema, infarction and haemorrhage in the surrounding brain parenchyma. The stroke caused by intracerebral haemorrhage is due to focal collection of blood within the brain parenchyma or ventricular system that is not caused by trauma. Haemorrhagic stroke can also occur due to sub arachnoid haemorrhage (SAH) [37].

The incidence of stroke during pregnancy including cerebral venous thrombosis ranges from 10 to 34/100,000 deliveries [38, 39]. In a large population based study in the USA, 2850 pregnancy related strokes were identified with a rate of 34.2/100,000 deliveries. The authors estimated a three fold increase in strokes in pregnant rather than non-pregnant women [39]. The incidence of a stroke during pregnancy and puerperium in this study was 39 per 100,000 deliveries. One of the most common risk factors for strokes in pregnancy, particularly postpartum, is preeclampsia/ eclampsia [39, 40]. A nationwide inpatient sample analysis reported that preeclampsia is associated with a 4-fold increase in stroke during pregnancy. Hypertension is associated with both ischemic and haemorrhagic strokes [28, 39]. In our study, the causes of neurological deficits and blindness included arterial infarcts in 30.2% of cases, intracerebral haemorrhage in 13.1% of cases and cerebral vein thrombosis in 10.5% of cases. PRES in 10.5% of cases and cerebral oedema in 18.4% of cases.

Arterial Ischemic Stroke

The arterial ischemic stroke in eclampsia is due to occlusion of a cerebral artery resulting in infarction of the central nervous system and can occur through multiple mechanisms. Preeclampsia/eclampsia related hypercoagulability and severe vasospasm cause hypoperfusion distal to the point of spasm, resulting in acute ischemic stroke [41]. Studies have shown that a history of migraines, particularly if associated with aura, increases the risk of acute ischemic stroke to 8- to 30-fold [42]. The overall incidence of ischemic stroke during pregnancy is low (3.5-5 per 100 000 pregnancies in the developed world), with the majority of these events occurring late in pregnancy and particularly in the postpartum period [43, 44]. In this study, 23 cases of arterial infarcts were diagnosed on neuro imaging, 12 (52.2%) cases occurred in the antepartum period and 11 (47.8%) in the postpartum period. Except for one case who had MRI, all the others were diagnosed by CT imaging. The CT scan imaging findings included focal loss of the normal borderline between the gray matter and white matter of brain and low attenuation. Hypoattenuation on CT is highly specific for irreversible ischemic brain damage if it is detected within first 6 hours. The loss of grey/white matter differentiation which evolves into reduced density is normally seen in an arterial supply territory, and is often associated with cerebral oedema. A high signal on conventional MR-sequences is comparable to hypodensity on CT. It is the result of irreversible injury with cell death [45]. Many studies have shown that the risk of stroke is high in the postpartum period. Kittner et al. showed that for cerebral infarction, the RR during pregnancy adjusted for age and race was 0.7 (95%CI 0.3 to 1.6), but it increased to 8.7 for the postpartum period (95%CI 4.6 to 16.7) [44]. However, in our study on logistic regression analysis, only diastolic BP was found to be a significant risk factor for the occurrence of arterial infarction. Patients with DBP greater than 110 were 3.29 times (aOR 3.29, 95% CI 1.14-9.52) more likely to develop arterial infarcts as compared to patients with DBP 80-110 mm of Hg. Reports from western countries have shown that most pregnancy related strokes are attributable to arterial occlusion [38, 44, 46]. Our study also showed that the majority of strokes were due to arterial infarcts. However, a previous Indian study by Srinivasan has shown that arterial infarcts occurred only in 6 of the 135 women with a stroke [32].

Stroke due to Intracerebral Haemorrhage

Intracerebral haemorrhage is a life threatening complication of eclampsia. Eclamptic women are prone to develop ICH as a result of severe hypertension [47]. The vascular pathophysiology of ICH in preeclampsia / eclampsia may be due to arteriolar dysfunction, with compromised autoregulation unable to compensate for acute hypertension which could be aggravated by preeclampsia-related coagulopathy [48]. Haemorrhage may occur following a rupture of a vessel or after infarction, either spontaneously or caused by antithrombotic or thrombolytic therapy. Haemorrhage after infarction ranges in severity from minor petechial bleeding to haemorrhage causing mass effect and secondary injury. This has been referred to as "haemorrhagic infarction" [49, 50]. Cerebral infarction transforming into a haemorrhagic infarction may be more common in young nulliparae who present with parietooccipital and temporal distribution of vasogenic oedema [29]. Witlin et al. have shown that cerebrovascular malformations are seen in 20% of patients with pregnancy related ICH [51]. Cerebral haemorrhage may be more common in older women with underlying chronic hypertension which can damage small or medium-sized cerebral arteries. The thalamus, cerebellum, and brain stem are the sites most frequently affected in such hypertensive intracerebral haemorrhage. In our analysis, there were no cases of hypertension with superimposed pre-eclampsia/eclampsia.

CT scan is almost always the first imaging modality used to assess patients with suspected intracranial haemorrhage. There is little difficulty in the diagnosis of cerebral haemorrhage as the acute blood is markedly hyperdense compared to brain parenchyma. In the acute setting, CT and MR imaging have extremely high sensitivity and specificity and have been shown to be 96% concordant with each other [52]. The risk factors independently associated with haemorrhagic stroke included pre-existing hypertension (OR 2.6; 95% CI 1.34–5.07), gestational hypertension (OR 2.41; 95% CI 1.62–3.59), and preeclampsia/eclampsia (OR 10.4; 95% CI 8.3–13.0) [53]. Data from the Nationwide Inpatient Sample examining women aged 15 to 44 showed that most cases of pregnancy-associated haemorrhagic strokes occurred postpartum and the authors have reported that haemorrhagic stroke is the most common stroke type associated with pregnant or postpartum women with preeclampsia/eclampsia [54]. Kittner et al. showed that for the occurrence of intracerebral haemorrhage, the adjusted RR was 2.5 during pregnancy (95%CI 1.0 to 6.4), but 28.3 for the postpartum period (95%CI 13.0 to 61.4) [44]. Our findings are similar to other authors' studies and by both univariate and multivariate models, timing of eclampsia was found to be a significant predictor of ICH and patients with postpartum eclampsia were 6.44 times (aOR 6.44, 95% CI 1.52-27.32) more likely to develop ICH as compared to patients with antepartum eclampsia. SBP was also found significant in the multivariate model. As compared to patients with SBP less than or equal to 160, patients with SBP greater than 160 were 5.75 times (aOR 5.75, 95% CI 1.31-25.19) more likely to develop ICH in the adjusted analysis. It is speculated that hypertension and coagulopathy increase the risk of haemorrhagic transformation in previously ischemic areas of the brain. In our study, among the 6 cases who developed HELLP syndrome, two of them had ICH.

Stroke due to Cerebral Venous Thrombosis (CVT)

Cerebral venous and sinus thrombosis (CVT) is a subtype of stroke which may result in ischemic and/or haemorrhagic complications. Pregnancy and the immediate postpartum period are associated with a significant increase in the risk of cerebral venous thrombosis [55]. Pregnancy induces a degree of physiologic hypercoagulability in order to prepare for delivery and reduce the chance of maternal haemorrhage. Normal pregnancy causes changes in the coagulation system that contribute to an increased risk of venous thrombotic events, including CVT, particularly in the puerperium [56]. In the setting of preeclampsia / eclampsia, there is hypercoagulability of blood, systemic inflammation, platelet activation, and endothelial injury, all of which predispose to thrombosis and increase the risk of CVT especially in the postpartum period [39]. Maternal hypertension was shown to increase the risk of CVT by an odds ratio of 1.9 [57]. Other genetic causes of hypercoagulability including antiphospholipid syndrome, prothrombin gene mutations, and factor V Leiden/MHTFR deficiency are associated with the development of CVT [58, 59]. Hyper-homocystinaemia, and sickle–cell disease may also contribute to the occurrence of CVT in pregnancy. Other contributing factors for the occurrence of venous thrombotic events are infection, caesarean section, obesity, prolonged bed rest, anaemia and dehydration in the postpartum period. These factors are seen commonly in developing countries [55]. In many patients, more than one risk factor may be present and a single causal mechanism for the occurrence of thrombosis may not be identified. Cerebral venous thrombosis (CVT) can involve the intracranial venous sinuses, the deep venous system, and cortical veins that drain into the major intracranial sinuses. In the early stages there is cortical vein thrombosis and later, sinuses are involved. The main sinuses affected by CVT are the superior sagittal sinus, and lateral sinuses. Occlusion of venous system leads to venous congestion, focal oedema, and the resultant venous stasis leads to tissue ischemia and infarction. In 10-15% of cases, due to the elevated venous and capillary pressure, secondary petechial or frank haemorrhage may occur within the brain parenchyma [60, 61, 62]. The overall risk of developing a CVT remains low in developed countries (11.6 per 100 000 pregnancies) [57]. CVT during pregnancy and puerperium is a common entity in India. Bansal et al. reported an incidence of 4.5 /10,000 obstetric admissions [63]. The high incidence of CVT in the Indian population may be due to sepsis, anaemia and the custom of withholding fluid in the postpartum period leading to dehydration. However, in our report, CVT contributed only to 19.5% of all cases of stroke. There were 8 cases where the neurological complications were due to CVT. Among these, 2 cases presented in the antepartum period and the other 6 cases manifested in the postpartum period. The case which occurred in the antepartum period was APLA positive. By both univariate and multivariate models, the timing of eclampsia was found to be significant predictor of CVT in this study. Patients with postpartum eclampsia were 9.59 times (aOR 9.59, 95% CI 2.00-46.08) more likely to develop CVT as compared to patients with antepartum eclampsia in the adjusted analysis. Though anaemia has been described as an important aetiological factor for the occurrence of CVT, both by univariate and multivariate analysis, anaemia was not found be a significant predictor of CVT in our analysis.

The clinical presentation related to CVT is quite variable and depends upon the territory of the affected vascular system. Most commonly, the superior sagittal and transverse sinuses are affected by and associated with headache, seizures, and papilledema if severe enough to cause increased intracranial pressures. Headache is the presenting symptom in 70-90% of cases. In the postpartum period, a headache is often mistaken for a post-dural puncture headache or migraine [39]. Caesarean section and infections, both of which are more common in women with preeclampsia, increase the risk of postpartum CVT [57]. In CVT, symptoms are caused by the obstruction of cortical veins and superior longitudinal sinus. This results in impaired CSF absorption, causing raised intra cranial pressure or obstruction of the draining veins resulting in venous congestion and cerebral infarction. There is also edema in the vicinity of an occluded sinus and/or tributary vein leading to visual disturbances and decreased levels of consciousness can occur. Occlusion of the deep cerebral veins involving the basal ganglia and thalamus may result in focal neurological findings such as hemiparesis or aphasia. Depending on the thrombosis of specific sinuses, the clinical presentation can vary. The cavernous sinus is less commonly affected and may present with cranial nerve deficits, headaches, proptosis, and painful opthalmoplegia related to increased pressure within the sinus and orbit. Involvement of the cranial nerve 5 or 6 can occur in thrombosis of the lateral sinus with extension to the superior or inferior petrosal sinus. Cranial nerves 9, 10, and 11 can be affected from extension of lateral sinus thrombosis into the jugular bulb [64, 65].

Non-contrast CT imaging which is often done in an ER setting, may reveal CVT but is less reliable than MRI. A contrast-enhanced CT head and CT-venography (CTV) may provide detailed visualization of the venous sinuses however, the use of contrast material would not be the first choice in the pregnant patient. Venous infarcts related to CVT do not occur in the typical distributions represented by arterial infarctions and this can be a clue that an underlying CVT is present. Magnetic resonance imaging of the brain is the best initial study to work up potential CVT in a pregnant patient as it does not require contrast administration and may also facilitate visualization of both the thrombus and the surrounding brain parenchyma

[66]. A rapid and reliable diagnosis of thrombo - occlusive disease is important because early therapy can prevent further complications of CVT. A CT scan remains the first imaging modality because of the easy availability and to exclude conditions such as intracerebral haemorrhage.

Posterior Reversible Encephalopathy Syndrome (PRES)

Besides ischemic and haemorrhagic strokes, in recent years Posterior Reversible Encephalopathy Syndrome (PRES) has been implicated as one of the important causes for neurological manifestations in eclampsia. It is also called reversible posterior leukoencephalopathy syndrome (RPLS). It is a neurological syndrome associated with a unique CT or MR imaging appearance. This disorder differs from ischemic or haemorrhagic stroke because it is associated with reversible vasogenic oedema seen on CT or MRI, usually in the occipital or parietal lobes. Pre-eclampsia is one of the important conditions associated with this syndrome. In PRES there is disruption of the blood-brain barrier due to hypertension induced capillary damage and immune mediated endothelial cell dysfunction. This leads to the extravasation of fluid into the perivascular space causing cerebral oedema [35]. The vasogenic edema and breakdown in blood brain barrier affect both cortical and subcortical structures and has a predilection for the parietal and occipital lobes. The characteristic imaging feature includes focal regions of symmetric edema in the posterior brain parenchyma [35, 67]. The area supplied by the posterior circulation is most vulnerable to breakthrough of the blood–brain barrier because of less sympathetic innervation and less ability for neurogenic response to increased blood pressure and there are rapid fluctuations in blood flow and water content of the brain. Though the parieto-occipital region is commonly involved, the lesions may extend to the brain stem, cerebellum, basal ganglia, and the more anterior brain regions, such as the frontal lobes. This syndrome may develop even with only mild hypertension in the presence of concomitant endothelial damage. Large changes in blood pressure (rather than the absolute blood pressure) can result in an imbalance of the capillary and cellular perfusion pressures, leading to vasogenic oedema [45, 68]. The most common clinical manifestations of PRES include headaches, confusion, seizures, and visual changes such as cortical blindness. In severe cases, PRES may result in coma, status epilepticus, and neurological deficits. In more severe cases it can lead to neurological morbidity or mortality due to ischemic stroke or haemorrhage [69]. In our study among the 8 cases who were diagnosed with PRES on neuroimaging, the clinical manifestations were cortical blindness in 1 case, facial palsy in 1 cases and aphasia in 6 cases. All patients recovered without residual deficits. Studies have shown that up to 98% of women with eclampsia have radiological evidence of PRES [70]. Recognizing PRES is important because the neurologic disorder is readily treatable by lowering blood pressure and correction of the underlying medical condition that contributed to the endothelial dysfunction. The treatment of PRES in the pregnant patient is similar to that of eclampsia using antihypertensives and anticonvulsants. Emergency delivery would be required in these patients [29, 71].

Visual Disturbances

The most common ocular complaint in pre-eclampsia/eclampsia is blurred vision which was seen in 36.8% of our patients. The major ocular complication seen in this study was blindness due to cortical blindness and retinal detachment. In the past, blindness was usually attributed to retinal abnormalities such as retinal detachment thrombosis of the central retinal artery, and retinal arteriolar vasospasm. With the availability of newer neuroimaging modalities, such as MRI, it is established that cerebral oedema, especially in the occipital region, and the region of lateral geniculate nuclei can result in transient blindness and is termed "cortical blindness." Transient cortical blindness is estimated to occur in about 15% of eclamptic women [14]. Acute onset of visual symptoms in pregnant women can be the first sign of pre-eclampsia [72]. Cortical blindness results from petechial haemorrhages and focal oedema in the parieto-occipital area affecting the ocular region. In our study, cortical blindness was seen in 2.4% of eclampsia cases. Chakravarty et al. reported 5 cases with visual disturbances among 19 eclampsia cases [73]. Blindness due to pre-eclampsia/eclampsia can occur at any period of gestation. In our analysis, in 13 of the 22 cases, cortical blindness manifested in the antepartum and intrapartum period and in 9 cases in the postpartum period. Blindness occurring in the antepartum period is an indication for terminating the pregnancy. In six cases where blindness occurred in the antepartum period, we have delivered them within 8 hours. Blurring of vision and intense headache preceded blindness in all the cases and these symptoms were seen 2-6 hours prior to the manifestation of blindness. Therefore, it is important for the clinicians to anticipate complications such as blindness and cerebro-vascular accidents in those presenting with intense headaches. There could be associated lesions at other sites of the brain as well. Manifestations of pyramidal dysfunction such as clonus, plantar extensor, hemiparesis/hemiplegia and aphasia have all been reported [74]. In our analysis, 6 patients also had neurological manifestations such as hemiparesis, hemiplegia and aphasia. The radiological findings in cortical blindness ranges from normal to widespread low density areas in the parieto-occipital region by CT scan. The MRI studies demonstrate high signal intensity areas related to focal cerebral oedema and ischemia [75]. Neuroimaging studies by Chakravarthy et al. have also shown that the visual cortex is affected by oedema, micro-infarction and micro-haemorrhages [73]. In our study, neuroimaging findings were reported normal in 8 cases, cerebral oedema in 10 cases, PRES in 1 case and arterial infarcts in 3 cases. Cortical blindness is generally reversible and permanent blindness from retinal vascular change is rare. Most pre-eclamptic women with cortical blindness recover vision over a period varying from 2 hours to 21 days [14]. Ozkan et al. have suggested that blindness in pre-eclampsia/eclampsia might be reversible, if the neuroimaging studies are associated with petechial haemorrhages, ischemia and focal oedema in the occipital cortex region [75]. In this study, recovery of vision occurred within 24 hours in 27.3% of cases and vision was recovered in all 22 cases within 10 days. Other than the effective treatment of pre-eclampsia/eclampsia and termination of pregnancy, no specific therapy is indicated in pre-eclamptic women who experience ocular changes. Retinal detachment is an unusual cause of visual loss in pre-eclampsia/eclampsia. Due to severe hypertension there is separation of the neurosensory retina from the pigmented retinal epithelium leading to visual loss. They tend to be bilateral, bullous, and associated with retinopathy changes. Management of retinal detachment in pre-eclampsia is conservative and involves treating the underlying condition. The prognosis is good and spontaneous resolution usually occurs with adequate control of BP and delivery. The finding of retinal detachment is an indication for terminating pregnancy.

Diagnosis

The initial task for the clinician is to distinguish real stroke from stroke mimics and, if real, to differentiate between ischemic and haemorrhagic events. The selection of the neuroimaging modality depends on the availability of the imaging technique, as rural hospitals and developing regions are less likely to have access to imaging, especially MRI. The critical nature of the patient should also be taken into consideration while deciding on the neuroimaging modality. An initial study with a non-contrast head computerized tomography (CT) with appropriate foetal shielding in antenatal mothers or a magnetic resonance imaging (MRI) of the brain greatly facilitates diagnosis with minimal risk to the foetus [76]. Computed tomography (CT) scanning, is more readily available in most medical centres than magnetic resonance imaging (MRI), and is usually able to exclude stroke mimics such as brain tumours and can differentiate brain ischemia from haemorrhage. The imaging modality available in our centres was CT scanning. However, three patients were referred to other centres for MRI studies. MRI is often the preferred imaging study for a pregnant patient as there is no radiation involved. A plain head CT scan, which is widely available, exposes the foetus to approximately 0.5cGy of radiation which is about 1% of the accepted threshold for cumulative foetal exposure [76]. If CT scanning is used in the antenatal period, care must be taken to shield the fetus from radiation exposure as much as possible. If MRI is available, it is extremely effective for the diagnosis of haemorrhage/ischemia or oedema in pre-eclampsia. It has been shown that CT can be entirely normal in 10-20% of cases with proven CVT [29]. In 13 of our patients, the CT imaging was reported normal in spite of the neurological manifestations. In these patients, MRI would probably have helped to identify the possible pathology.

Management

The initial management is to control convulsions, reduce blood pressure and intracranial pressure and resort to early delivery. Further management depends on the findings on neuro-imaging studies. Though there have been reports of using tissue plasminogen activator (tPA) in the management of ischemic stroke, studies in the pregnant population are sparse. The major side effect of tPA in adults is haemorrhage, including intracerebral haemorrhage. There is also concern that the use of tPA on the pregnant patient may lead to placental abruption, abortion, and preterm delivery. However, with the available data, the maternal mortality is 1%, foetal loss 6%, and preterm delivery is 6% [77]. Ischaemic stroke is generally treated by anticoagulation with unfractionated or low molecular weight heparin in our units. Following delivery, it is recommended to use warfarin for 3 to 6 months followed by repeat imaging [78]. Though hypertension may be the cause of arterial infarct, it is important to evaluate for an underlying hypercoagulable state so as to take preventive measures. Low dose aspirin has been recommended for future prevention. Management of ICH involves the use of antihypertensives, correction of coagulopathies, antiseizure medications and drugs are given to reduce the intracranial pressure. Blood and blood products are also given to replace the clotting factors. There have been reports on neurosurgical decompression of ICH [47]. Labetalol has been suggested as the first-line agent for hypertension accompanying stroke in preeclampsia as it lowers the cerebral perfusion pressure without affecting cerebral perfusion [79]. In patients with CVT, measures are taken to control the hypertension, seizures and raised intracranial pressure. Anticoagulants are given to prevent the extension of thrombus and to promote early recanalization. During pregnancy unfractionated heparin is used at sufficient dose to keep APTT 1.8-2 times the control. Following delivery, warfarin is used for anticoagulation which is generally continued for a 3 to 6 month period with repeat imaging to establish the status of recanalization [80]. In patients who are not improving with systemic anticoagulation therapy, interventional therapy utilizing thrombolytics or mechanical embolectomy are considered [81]. Liberal use of imaging modalities and early recourse to anticoagulation therapy in indicated cases will considerably reduce permanent sequelae such as epilepsy, residual focal neurological deficit and optic atrophy.

Prognosis

Globally, 42,000 deaths occur every year due to hypertensive disorders of pregnancy which accounts for 14% of all maternal deaths [4]. Our findings are similar to that of global rates and for the study period 14.75% of maternal deaths were reported due to pre-eclampsia/eclampsia/ hypertension. The incidence of eclampsia reported by Rabiu et al. from Nigeria was 2.8% with the case fatality rate of 19.4% [82]. Even in developed countries, hypertensive disorders account for a significant proportion of maternal deaths: in the UK, between 2006 and 2008, 18% of direct maternal deaths were due to pre-eclampsia/eclampsia. [83]. Though eclampsia leads to multiorgan dysfunction, there is predominant cerebro-vascular involvement which could be the direct mechanism of death in nearly 40% of patients. In the UK, among the 19 maternal deaths between 2006 and 2008 attributable to preeclampsia, nine (47%) occurred as a result of intracerebral bleeds [83]. However in developing countries like India, pulmonary oedema is reported to be the most common cause of death in eclampsia [8]. Our study also showed that pulmonary oedema was the most common mode of death, followed by CVA. The case fatality rate in this study was 14.5%. Among the 11 deaths that occurred due to neurological complications of eclampsia, 10 deaths were due to ICH, a fatality rate of 100% for ICH. At the time of admission, these patients were admitted in the stage of coma with very high levels of systolic and diastolic blood pressure. Early referral, effective anti hypertensive therapy and timely intervention and delivery of pre-eclampsia cases would have prevented or reduced the severity of these catastrophic events. In a 30 year study from UK, ICH was the single greatest cause of maternal death from stroke [84]. Mortality related to CVT is estimated at 9% and is primarily due to secondary intracerebral haemorrhage [85]. There were no deaths due to CVT in our study.

Long Term Consequences

There is increasing evidence that previously preeclamptic women face increased lifetime risks of ill health, predominantly due to cardiovascular events and metabolic disease. Recent data demonstrate the long-term persistence of brain white matter lesions possibly incurred at the time of eclamptic convulsions [86]. Even more concerning are recent epidemiologic data to suggest profound long-term cerebrovascular consequences, including a 3- to 5-fold increased risk for death from stroke in previously pre-eclamptic women [87[. Increased risk of Alzheimer's disease, vascular dementia and cognitive impairment have also been demonstrated [88].

Prevention

The recognition and prompt treatment of severe hypertension in pregnancy remains the mainstay of preventing neurological complications and death related to eclampsia. Guidelines generally recommend immediate antihypertensive therapy for blood pressures consistently equal to or greater than a systolic of 160 mmHg and/or diastolic of 110 mmHg, equating to a mean arterial pressure (MAP) of around 130 mmHg [89]. However, a significant proportion of patients may sustain an intracerebral bleed at MAPs lower than 130 mmHg [28] and there is evolving evidence to suggest that the rapidity of change in blood pressure and the absolute level of systolic blood pressure may be of greater clinical relevance. In general, blood pressure needs to be reduced to a safe range to avoid loss of cerebral autoregulation. In 2014, the American Heart Association and the American Stroke Association have released guidelines on stroke prevention in women. The guideline classifies hypertension in pregnancy as mild (diastolic BP-90-99 mm Hg or systolic BP 140-149 mm Hg), moderate (diastolic BP -100-109 mm Hg or systolic 150-159 mm Hg) or severe (diastolic BP > 110 mm Hg or systolic > 160 mm Hg). The recommendations are to control moderate and severe hypertension with safe and effective antihypertensive medications such as methyldopa, labetalol, and nifedipine. The goal is to maintain systolic BP between 130 and 155 mm Hg and diastolic BP between 80 and 105 mm Hg [90]. Besides controlling hypertension, prevention and treatment of eclamptic seizures with parenteral magnesium sulphate is also important to prevent the development of PRES and haemorrhagic stroke [91]. The proposed progression from arterial and venous infarctions to haemorrhagic infarctions may have important therapeutic implications. Early institution of anticoagulant therapy in those with arterial and venous infarctions may prevent the haemorrhagic complications which has the worst prognosis. However, cases should be carefully handled to avoid iatrogenic induction of ICH. It is also important to be aware of atypical presentation of eclampsia, so that delay in treating these patients can be avoided. In the postpartum period, dizziness, sudden confusion, loss of coordination, sudden, severe headache and difficulty seeing in one or both eyes should alert the physician as to the possibility impending neurological complications. In recent years, vitamin D deficiency has emerged as an important potentially modifiable risk factor for both preeclampsia and stroke. Women who are deficient in vitamin D before or during pregnancy should be identified and corrected [92].

CONCLUSION

This highlights the importance of creating awareness among the public to seek early medical attention as well as educating health care professionals and para-medical staffs in timely identification and treatment of pre-eclampsia through continuing medical education and the use of clinical guidelines for management.

While treating cases of pre-eclampsia and eclampsia, clinicians must be vigilant and investigate CNS complaints with imaging studies so as to identify evolving CNS pathology. As this study has shown that postpartum eclampsia is a significant risk factor for the occurrence of neurological complications, more vigilance is required in the first two weeks after delivery. Clinicians should be aware of the ocular manifestations and careful ophtholomological and neurological evaluation should be carried out along with neuro-imaging studies to ascertain the various causes of blindness in pregnancy. The prognosis is usually good with effective treatment of pre-eclampsia/eclampsia along with termination of pregnancy. The finding of papilledema on fundoscopy is an emergency, and urgent measures should be taken to identify and treat the cause for increased ICT. The limitations of this study are that this is a retrospective analysis of case records and prospective studies may throw more light onto the diagnosis, management and prevention of these conditions. Except in few cases, CT imaging was the only imaging modality that was available and for the immediate management of ICH, neurosurgical support was not available during the study period.

ACKNOWLEDGMENTS

The authors thank the Heads of Govt. Hospital for Women and Children and Meenakshi Medical College Hospital and Research Institute for giving us permission to conduct this study. Our sincere thanks are due to Mr. Ananta Ghimire, Biostatistician from Beyond P Value for his excellent statistical support. We are thankful to Mr M Balaji Prabhu for his support in preparing and formatting the figures.

DISCLOSURE

The authors declare no conflicts of interest and no financial support was received for this study.

REFERENCES

[1] Aagaard-Tillery KM., Belfort MA. (2005) Eclampsia: morbidity, mortality, and management. *Clin Obstet Gynecol.* 48(1):12–23.

[2] Sibai BM., Stella CL. (2009) Diagnosis and management of atypical preeclampsia-eclampsia. *Am J Obstet Gynecol.* 200(5):481.e1-7.

[3] Kodandapani S and Pai Ah. (2018) Atypical Preeclampsia: A Review. *J Gynecol Women's Health* 12(5): JGWH.MS.ID.555849.

[4] Say L., Chou D., Gemmill A., Tuncalp O., Moller AB., Daniels J., Gülmezoglu AM., Temmerman M., Alkema L. (2014). Global causes of maternal death: a WHO systematic analysis. *The Lancet* Global Health; 2: e 323-33.

[5] World Health Organization. Trends in maternal mortality: 1990 to 2015. Estimates by WHO, UNICEF, UNFPA, *The World Bank and the United Nations Population Division.* Geneva: World Health Organization; 2015. http://apps.who.int/iris/bitstream/10665/194254/1/9789241565141_eng.pdf?ua=1. Accessed on 14.02.2021.

[6] Knight M., Nair M., Tuffnell D., Kenyon S., Shakespeare J., Brocklehurst P., Kurinczuk JJ. (2016) *Saving lives, improving mothers' care—surveillance of maternal deaths in the UK 2012–14 and lessons learned to inform maternity care from the UK and Ireland Confidential Enquiries into Maternal Deaths and Morbidity 2009–14.* Oxford: Nuffield Department of Population Health.

[7] Micheal BB. (2000) Eclampsia. *Emer Med J.* 74:1–10.
[8] Das R and Biswas S. (2015). Eclapmsia: The Major Cause of Maternal Mortality in Eastern India. *Ethiop J Health Sci.* 25(2): 111–116.
[9] Tuffnell DJ., Jankowicz D., Lindow SW., Lyons G., Mason GC., Russell IF., Walker JJ. (2005) Outcomes of severe preeclampsia / eclampsia in Yorkshire 1999/2003. *BJOG;* 112 (7):875-880.
[10] Lewis, G (ed) 2007. The Confidential Enquiry into Maternal and Child Health (CEMACH). Saving Mothers' Lives: reviewing maternal deaths to make motherhood safer - 2003-2005. *The Seventh Report on Confidential Enquiries into Maternal Deaths in the United Kingdom.* London: CEMACH.
[11] Miller EC. (2019) Preeclampsia and Cerebrovascular Disease. *The Maternal Brain at Risk Hypertension.* 74:5–13.
[12] Miller EC., Gatollari HJ., Too G., Boehme AK., Leffert L., Marshall RS., Elkind MSV., Willey JZ. (2017) Risk Factors for Pregnancy-Associated Stroke in Women with Preeclampsia. *Stroke.* 48(7):1752-1759.
[13] *World Health Organization (WHO)* Definition of Stroke - Public Health, 2020- https://www.publichealth.com.ng/world-health-organization-who-definition-of-stroke. Accessed on 23/01/2021.
[14] Cunningham FG., Fernandez CO., Hernandez C. (1995) Blindness associated with preeclampsia and eclampsia. *Am J Obstet Gynecol.* 172:1291-1298.
[15] IBM Corp. Released 2013. *IBM SPSS Statistics for Windows, Version 22.0.* Armonk, NY: IBM Corp.
[16] Steegers EA., von Dadelszen P., Duvekot JJ., and Pijnenborg R. (2010) "Pre-eclampsia," *The Lancet.* 376: 631–644.
[17] Abalos E., Cuesta C., Grosso AL., Chou D., Say L. (2013) Global and regional estimates of preeclampsia and eclampsia: a systematic review. *Eur J Obstet Gynecol Reprod Biol.* 170(1):1–7.
[18] Saftlas AF., Olson DR., Franks AL., Atrash HK., Pokras R. (1990) Epidemiology of preeclampsia and eclampsia in the United States 1979-1986. *Am J Obstet Gynecol* 163:460-465.

[19] Zwart JJ., Richters A., Ory F., de Vries Johanna IP., Bloemenkamp KWM., van Roosmalen J. (2008) Eclampsia in the Netherlands. *Obstet Gynecol* 112:820-827.

[20] Knight M: (2005) Eclampsia in the United Kingdom. *Br J Obstet Gynaecol* 2007; 114:1072-1078.

[21] Abalos E., Cuesta C., Carroli G., Qureshi Z., Widmer M., Vogel JP., Souza JP. (2014) Pre-eclampsia, eclampsia and adverse maternal and perinatal outcomes: a secondary analysis of the World Health Organization Multi Country Survey on Maternal and New Born Health. *BJOG*. 121(Suppl 1):14–24.

[22] Recent Report on FOGSI-GESTOSIS-ICOG Hypertensive Disorders in *Pregnancy (HDP) Good Clinical Practice Recommendations 2019*. https://www.fogsi.org/wp-content/uploads/gcpr/hdp-fogsi-gestosis-icog.

[23] Shanthirani B., Moogambigai K. (2016) Acute Neurologiclal Complications in Peripartum Period: A Retrospective Study. *Int J Sci Stud* 4 (4): 111-113.

[24] FAl-Hayali RM., Al-Habbo DJ., Hammo M K. (2008) Peripartum neurological emergencies in a Critical Care Unit. *Neurosciences* 13(2): 155-160.

[25] Mattar F., Sibai BM. (2000) Eclampsia. VIII. Risk factors for maternal morbidity. *Am J Obstet Gynecol*. 182 (2): 307–312.

[26] Douglas KA., Redman CWG. (1994) Eclampsia in the United Kingdom. *BMJ*. 309: 1395–1400.

[27] Mirza A. (2006) Posterior reversible encephalopathy syndrome: a variant of hypertensive encephalopathy. *J Clin Neurosci*. 13 (5): 590–595.

[28] Martin JN., Thigpen BD., Moore RC., Rose CH., Cushman J., and May W. (2005) "Stroke and severe preeclampsia and eclampsia: a paradigm shift focusing on systolic blood pressure," *Obstetrics and Gynecology*. 105 (2): 246–254.

[29] Zeeman GG, (2009) "Neurologic complications of pre-eclampsia," *Seminars in Perinatology*, 33(3): 166–172.

[30] Leszek M., Lech R. (2012) Acute cortical blindness in preeclampsia-- a case of reversible posterior encephalopathy syndrome. *Ginekol Pol* 83: 469-472.
[31] Bakhda RN. (2015) Clinical assessment of retinopathy post management of pregnancy induced hypertension. *International Journal of Medicine and Public Health*. 5 (3): 205-207.
[32] Srinivasan K. (1983) Cerebral venous and arterial thrombosis in pregnancy and puerperium – A study of 135 patients. *Angiology*. 34(11):731-746.
[33] Busija DW., Heistad DD. (1984) Factors involved in the physiological regulation of the cerebral circulation. *Rev Physiol Biochem Pharmacol*. 101: 161–211.
[34] Cunningham F. (2010) *Pregnancy Hypertension. In Williams Obstetrics 23rd ed. Eds.* Cunningham F., Leveno K, Bloom S. et al. New York. McGraw-Hill 2010, 713-714.
[35] Cipolla MJ. (2007) Cerebrovascular Function in Pregnancy and Eclampsia. *Hypertension*. 50:14–24.
[36] Prout, RE., Tuckey JP., Giffen NJ. (2007) Reversible posterior leucoencephalopathy syndrome in a peripartum patient. *International Journal of Obstetric Anesthesia*, 16(1): 74 – 76.
[37] Ralph L. Sacco, Scott E. Kasner, Joseph P. Broderick, Louis R. Caplan, JJ. Connors, Antonio Culebras, Mitchell SV. Elkind, Mary G. George, Allen D. Hamdan. (2013) An Updated Definition of Stroke for the 21st Century. *Stroke*. 44:2064–2089.
[38] Jaigobin C and Silver FL. (2000) "Stroke and Pregnancy," *Stroke*, 31(12): 2948–2951.
[39] James AH., Bushnell CD., Jamison MG., Myers ER. (2005) "Incidence and risk factors for stroke in pregnancy and the puerperium," *Obstetrics and Gynecology*. 106(3): 509–516.
[40] Lanska DJ and Kryscio RJ. (1998) "Stroke and intracranial venous thrombosis during pregnancy and puerperium," *Neurology*. 51(6): 1622–1628.
[41] Fugate JE., Wijdicks EF., Parisi JE., Kallmes DF., Cloft HJ., Flemming KD., Giraldo EA., Rabinstein AA. (2012). Fulminant

postpartum cerebral vasoconstriction syndrome. *Arch Neurol.* 69:111–117.

[42] Wabnitz A, Bushnell C. (2015) Migraine, cardiovascular disease, and stroke during pregnancy: systematic review of the literature. *Cephalalgia.* 35:132–139.

[43] Feske S. Stroke in pregnancy. (2007) *Semin Neurol.* 27(5):442–452

[44] Kittner SJ., Stern BJ., Feeser BR., Hebel JR., Nagey DA., Buchholz DW. (1996) Pregnancy and the risk of stroke. *N Engl J Med* 335(11): 768 – 774.

[45] Schwartz RB., Feske SK., Polak JF., DeBirolami U., Iaia A., Beckner KM., Bravo SM., Klufas RA., Chai RYC., Repke JT. (2000) Preeclampsia-eclampsia: clinical and neuroradiographic correlates and insights into the pathogenesis of hypertensive encephalopathy. *Radiology.* 217:371-6.

[46] Sharshar T., Lamy C., Mas JL. (1995). Incidence and causes of strokes associated with pregnancy and puerperium. *Stroke* 26 (6): 930-936.

[47] Dai X., Diamond JA. (2007) Intracerebral haemorrhage: A life threatening complication of hypertension during pregnancy. *J Clin Hypertens.* 9 (11): 897-900.

[48] Johnson AC., Cipolla MJ. (2018) Impaired function of cerebral parenchymal arterioles in experimental preeclampsia. *Microvasc Res.* 119:64–72.

[49] The National Institute of Neurological Disorders and Stroke rt-PA Stroke Study Group. Tissue plasminogen activator for acute ischemic stroke. (1995) *N Engl J Med.* 333:1581–1587.

[50] International Stroke Trial Collaborative Group. The International Stroke Trial (IST): a randomised trial of aspirin, subcutaneous heparin, both, or neither among 19435 patients with acute ischaemic stroke. *Lancet.* 1997; 349:1569–1581.

[51] Witlin AG., Mattar F., Sibai BM. (2000) Postpartum stroke: a twenty year experience. *Am J Obstet Gynecol.* 183(1): 83-88.

[52] Kidwell CS., Chalela JA., Saver JL., Starkman S., Hill MD., Demchuk AM., Butman JA., Patronas N., Alger JR., Latour LL.,

Luby ML., Baird AE., Leary MC., Tremwel M., Ovbiagele B., Fredieu A., Suzuki S., Villablanca JP., Davis S., Dunn B., Todd JW., Ezzeddine MA., Haymore J., Lynch JK., Davis L., Warach S. (2004) Comparison of MRI and CT for detection of acute intracerebral hemorrhage. *JAMA*. 292:1823–1830.

[53] Jeng S., Tang SC., and Yip PK. (2004) "Stroke in women of reproductive age: comparison between stroke related and unrelated to pregnancy," Journal of the Neurological Sciences. 221(1-2): 25–29.

[54] Bateman BT., H. Schumacher HC., C. D. Bushnell CD., Pile-Spellman JP., Simpson LL., Sacco RL., Berman MF. (2006). "Intracerebral hemorrhage in pregnancy: frequency, risk factors, and outcome," *Neurology*, vol. 67, no. 3, pp. 424–429.

[55] Ferro J., Canhão P., Stam J., Bousser M., Barinagarrementeria F., Investigators I. (2004) Prognosis of cerebral vein and dural sinus thrombosis: results of the International Study on Cerebral Vein and Dural Sinus Thrombosis (ISCVT). *Stroke*; 35(3):664–670.

[56] Kamel H., Navi BB., Sriram N., Hovsepian DA., Devereux RB., Elkind MS. (2014) Risk of a thrombotic event after the 6-week postpartum period. *N Engl J Med*. 370:1307–1315.

[57] Lanska DJ., Kryscio RJ. (2000) Risk factors for peripartum and postpartum stroke and intracranial venous thrombosis. *Stroke*; 31: 1274-1282.

[58] Treadwell S., Thanvi B., Robinson T. (2008) Stroke in pregnancy and the puerperium. *Postgrad Med J*. 84(991):238–245.

[59] Dentali F., Crowther M., Ageno W. (2006) Thrombophilic abnormalities, oral contraceptives, and risk of cerebral vein thrombosis: a meta-analysis. *Blood*. 107(7):2766–2773.

[60] Cumurciuc R., Crassard I., Sarov M., Valade D., Bousser MG. (2005) Headache as the only neurological sign of cerebral venous thrombosis: a series of 17 cases. *J Neurol Neurosurg Psychiatry*. 76:1084–1087.

[61] Pfefferkorn T., Crassard I., Linn J., Dichgans M., Boukobza M., Bousser MG. (2009) Clinical features, course and outcome in deep

cerebral venous system thrombosis: an analysis of 32 cases. *J Neurol.* 256:1839–1845.

[62] Oppenheim C., Domigo V., Gauvrit JY., Lamy C., Mackowiak-Cordoliani MA., Pruvo JP., Méder JF. (2005) Subarachnoid hemorrhage as the initial presentation of dural sinus thrombosis. *AJNR Am J Neuroradiol.* 26:614–617.

[63] Bansal BC., Gupta RR., Prakash C. (1980) Stroke during pregnancy and puerperium in young females below the age of 40 years as a result of cerebral venous/venous sinus thrombosis. *Jpn Heart J.* 21: 171-183.

[64] Stam J. (2005) Thrombosis of the cerebral veins and sinuses. *N Engl J Med.* 352:1791–1798.

[65] Damak M., Crassard I., Wolff V., Bousser MG. (2009) Isolated lateral sinus thrombosis: a series of 62 patients. *Stroke*; 40:476–481.

[66] Selim M., Caplan LR. (2008) Radiological diagnosis of cerebral venous thrombosis. *Front Neurol Neurosci.* 23:96–111.

[67] Hinchey J., Chaves C., Appignani B., Breen J., Pao L., Wang A., Pessin MS., Lamy C., Mas JL., Caplan LR. (1996). A reversible posterior leukoencephalopathy syndrome. *N Engl J Med.* 334(8):494–500.

[68] Lee VH., Wijdicks EFM., Manno EM., Rabinstein AA. (2008) "Clinical spectrum of reversible posterior leukoencephalopathy syndrome," *Archives of Neurology.* 65(2) 205–210.

[69] Fugate JE., Claassen DO., Cloft HJ., Kallmes DF., Kozak OS., Rabinstein AA. (2010) Posterior reversible encephalopathy syndrome: associated clinical and radiologic findings. *Mayo Clin Proc.* 85(5):427–432.

[70] Brewer J., Owens MY., Wallace K., Reeves AA., Morris R., Khan M., LaMarca B., Martin JN. (2013) Posterior reversible encephalopathy syndrome in 46 of 47 patients with eclampsia. *Am J Obstet Gynecol.* 208:468.e1–468.e6.

[71] Duley L., Henderson-Smart DJ., Chou D. (2010) Magnesium sulphate versus phenytoin for eclampsia. *Cochrane Database Syst Rev.* 2010;10:CD000128.

[72] Roos NM., Wiegman MJ., Jansonius NM., Zeeman GG. (2012) Visual disturbances in (pre) eclampsia. *Obstet Gynecol Surv.* 67 (4): 242-50.
[73] Chakravarty A and S D Chakraborti SD. (2002) The Neurology of Eclampsia: Some observations. *Neurology India* 50: 128-134.
[74] Hanswald M. Cortical blindness and late postpartum eclampsia. (1987) *Am J Emer Med* 5: 130-2.
[75] Ozkan SO., Korbeyli B., Bese T., Eret CT. (2009) Acute cortical blindness complicating pregnancy. *Anesth Analg.* 91: 609-11.
[76] Dineen R., Banks A., Lenthall R. (2005) Imaging of acute neurological conditions in pregnancy and the puerperium. *Clin Radiol.* 60(11):1156–1170.
[77] Murugappan A., Coplin W., Al-Sadat A., McAllen KJ., Schwamm LH., Wechsler LR., Kidwell CS, Saver JL, Starkman S., Gobin YP., Duckwiler G., Krueger M., Rordorf G., Broderick JP., Tietjen GE., Levine SR. (2006) Thrombolytic therapy of acute ischemic stroke during pregnancy. *Neurology.* 66(5):768–770.
[78] Hirsh J., Fuster V., Ansell J., Halperin JL. (2003) American Heart Association/American College of Cardiology Foundation guide to warfarin therapy. *J Am Coll Cardiol.* 41(9):1633–1652
[79] Belfort MA., Tooke-Miller C., Allen JC., Jr., Dizon-Townson D., Varner MA. (2002) Labetalol decreases cerebral perfusion pressure without negatively affecting cerebral blood flow in hypertensive gravidas. *Hypertension in Pregnancy.* 21(3):185–197.
[80] Bates SM., Greer IA., Pabinger I., Sofaer S., Hirsh J. (2008) Venous thromboembolism, thrombophilia, antithrombotic therapy, and pregnancy: American College of Chest Physicians Evidence-Based Clinical Practice Guidelines (8th Edition). *Chest.* 133(6 suppl):844S–886S
[81] Medel R., Monteith SJ., Crowley RW., Dumont AS. (2009) A review of therapeutic strategies for the management of cerebral venous sinus thrombosis. *Neurosurg Focus.* 27(5):E6.
[82] Rabiu KA., Adewunmi AA., Ottun TA., Akinlusi FM., Adebanjo AA., Alausa TG. (2018) Risk factors for maternal mortality

associated with eclampsia presenting at a Nigerian tertiary hospital. *Int J Womens Health.* 10:715-721.

[83] Centre for Maternal and Child Enquiries (CMACE). Saving mothers' lives: reviewing maternal deaths to make motherhood safer: 2006–2008. The eighth report of the confidential enquiries into maternal deaths in the United Kingdom. *British Journal of Obstetrics and Gynaecology.* 2011;118(supplement 1):1–203.

[84] Foo L., Bewley S., Rudd. (2013) Maternal death from stroke: a thirty year national retrospective review. *European Journal of Obstetrics & Gynecology and Reproductive Biology.* 171(2): 266-270.

[85] Cantu C., Barinagarrementeria F. (1993) Cerebral venous thrombosis associated with pregnancy and puerperium. Review of 67 cases. *Stroke.* 24(12):1880–1884.

[86] Aukes, A., de Groot, J., Aarnoudse J., and Zeeman G. (2009). Brain lesions several years after eclampsia. *Am J Obstet Gynecol.* 200(5), 504.e1-504.e5.

[87] Wilson BJ., Watson MS., Prescott GJ, Sarah S., Campbell DM, Philip H. (2003) Hypertensive diseases of pregnancy and risk of hypertension and stroke in later life: Results from cohort study. *Br Med J* 326:845.

[88] Debette S., Markus HS. (2010) The clinical importance of white matter hyperintensities on brain magnetic resonance imaging: systematic review and meta-analysis. *The British Medical Journal.* 341, article c3666.

[89] National Institute for Health and Clinical Excellence. *NICE clinical guideline 107: hypertension in pregnancy—the management of hypertensive disorders during pregnancy.* London, UK, 2011.

[90] Bushnell C., Mc Cullough LD., Award IA., Chireau MV., N. Fedder WN., Furie KL et al. (2014)Guidelines for the prevention of stroke in women: A statement for healthcare professionals from the American Heart Association/American Stroke Association. *Stroke.* 45:1545-1588.

[91] Sibai BM. (2004). Magnesium sulfate prophylaxis in preeclampsia: Lessons learned from recent trials. *Am J Obstet Gynecol.* 190:1520-1526.

[92] Bodnar LM., Catov JM., Simhan HN., Holick MF., Powers RW., and Roberts JM. (2007). "Maternal vitamin D deficiency increases the risk of preeclampsia," *Journal of Clinical Endocrinology and Metabolism*, 92 [9] 3517–3522.

In: Eclampsia
Editor: Sharon Wright

ISBN: 978-1-53619-574-3
© 2021 Nova Science Publishers, Inc.

Chapter 2

PRE-ECLAMPSIA: IT'S ALL ABOUT POTASSIUM

Fred Chasalow[*], *PhD*

IOMA LLC, Department of Laboratory Sciences,
VA Medical Center, San Francisco, CA, US

ABSTRACT

Pre-eclampsia is a risk factor for life-threatening hypertension during pregnancy. Although the symptoms of pre-eclampsia are well known, their underlying biochemistry is not understood. This chapter describes the discovery of phosphoester steroid conjugates and proposes a role for them in pre-eclampsia. The newly discovered steroids are unique in two ways: (a) each steroid is a phosphoester and (b) each steroid has more than 21 carbon atoms. Prior to this discovery, no steroids were known with either feature. None of the newly discovered steroids bind to nuclear receptors. Some of the newly discovered hormones are spiral lactones and function as potassium sparing hormones, just like spironolactone or digoxin. We propose that spiral steroids have a key role in pre-eclampsia and may account for the increased, long-term risk of renal and cardiac diseases in affected patients. This chapter has four parts: (a) isolation,

---

[*] Corresponding Author's E-mail: fchasalow@gmail.com.

structure, and biosynthesis, (b) evidence for function, (c) biological role and function during pregnancy and (d) proposes how the spiral lactones lead to life-threatening hypertension and to the long-term consequences of pre-eclampsia.

Keywords: spiral steroids, potassium sparing hormones, pre-eclampsia, mammalian cardiotonic steroids, DLM, Ionotropin

1. INTRODUCTION

1.1. Discovery

In 2018, we reported isolation of a novel candidate for the endogenous mammalian cardiotonic steroid and selected *Ionotropin* as its name. Ionotropin is a phosphocholine ester of a steroid with a spiral lactone E-ring. The discovery also included three precursors. These made it possible to identify a biosynthetic pathway. Ionotropin and 5-dehydro-Ionotropin both cross-react with digoxin-specific antibodies (DLM).

1.2. Function of Ionotropin

Most steroids with lactone E-rings (digoxin, ouabain, marinobufagenin, spironolactone, Ionotropin etc.) function as potassium sparing diuretics and are digoxin-like materials (DLM). No other endogenous mammalian potassium sparing hormones have been described.

1.3. Regulatory Background

Pre-eclampsia is a syndrome characterized by hypertension and proteinuria. Typically, the symptoms develop during the second half of gestation and, in some women, the syndrome becomes life threatening. The

FDA has not approved any diagnostic method for pre-eclampsia and without a diagnostic method, investigators cannot identify risk factors or a useful therapeutic approach.

1.4. Pilot Study

Global Alliance for the Prevention of Prematurity and Stillbirth (GAPPS) provided 40 serum samples from pregnant women of 24-26 weeks of gestational age: 20 samples from normotensive women and 20 samples from women with pre-eclampsia. Each sample was analyzed by mass spectroscopy for the concentration of each of the steroid phosphocholine esters. There was no difference in Ionotropin or other DLM levels between the two groups. However, two precursors were elevated significantly in serum from the patients with pre-eclampsia when compared to levels in normotensive women of the same gestational age.

1.5. Theory

In some pregnant women, fetal potassium is inadequate. In the second trimester, high maternal levels of the spiral steroid precursors are converted to spiral steroids by the fetal-placental unit. These function as potassium sparing hormones. We characterize the maternal response (hypertension and proteinuria) to a mild, continuous elevation of the spiral steroids as pre-eclampsia, with symptoms similar to an overdose of ouabain or spironolactone. At the time of parturition, most infants have cord spiral steroid levels 10 times that of normal adults. Apparently, this is one of the key fetal processes in preparing for childbirth. Premature development of hyper-spirolemia, made possible by second trimester elevated levels of precursors, may be the ultimate cause of the life-threatening hypertension that occurs during the third trimester. There may be other mechanisms that lead to pre-eclampsia.

2. DISCOVERY OF CARDIOTONIC STEROIDS

In the 1950s, Szent-Gyorgyi speculated that digoxin was not really a novel drug but was a substitute for an endogenous hormone [1]. The first step in the isolation of the proposed hormone was the development of an immunoassay for digoxin [2]. The assay showed that some patients actually had high serum levels of "digoxin" prior to the initiation of digoxin therapy. In fact, on the basis of immunoassay results, several nurses were accused of 'killing' newborn infants by administering digoxin [3]. The unknown, endogenous cardiotonic glycoside was designated as a Digoxin-Like Material (DLM).

2.1. First Candidate

In 1991, Hamlyn proposed that the endogenous cardiotonic steroid (DLM) was ouabain [4]. The basis for this suggestion was his isolation of 13 µg of 'ouabain' from 80 liters of human plasma, equivalent to 0.16 ng/ml. The strongest part of the data was his suggestion that the H-NMR spectrum obtained on the purified material was identical to the spectrum of authentic ouabain. However, (1) ouabain has a 21-hydroxyl group included as part of its lactone ring but patients with 21-hydroxylase deficiency had DLM in their serum [5]; (2) many of the hydrogen atoms in ouabain would have similar shifts to hydrogens in similar positions in many steroids, and (3) the glycoside component of ouabain, rhamnose, is not ordinarily isolated from mammals [6]. Further, Baecher, with an ultra-high sensitivity LC-MS assay, that could detect 2 pg/ml, could not confirm the presence of ouabain in human serum [7].

2.2. Our Candidate

In 2018, we reported isolation of a novel candidate for the endogenous mammalian cardiotonic steroid and selected *Ionotropin* as its name [8]. We identified three families characterized by the number of carbon atoms in the steroid; at least one member of each family is a spiral lactone. Spiral steroid lactones had not previously been reported in any animal. In brief, Ionotropin differs from plant cardiotonic glycosides in three ways: (1) rather than a glycoside, it is a phosphocholine ester; (2) the steroid portion had not been described previously; and (3) no one has proposed that cardiotonic steroids specifically function as potassium sparing hormones.

2.3. Nomenclature of Spiral Steroids

In total, our laboratory has identified the phosphoesters of 14 different steroids. No endogenous steroid phosphoesters and none of these steroids were known prior to our investigations. The compounds fit into four families, distinguished by the number of carbon atoms – 21, 23, 24 or 25 – in the steroid. Estrogens, androgens, progestogens, glucocorticoids and mineralocorticoids would not be included in any of these families. Except for the two steroids with 21 carbon atoms, there are no trivial, recognized names for any of the other steroids.

When the classical steroids were discovered, laboratories used mobility on thin layer or paper chromatography to identify individual steroids. However, as all methods were not exactly equivalent, the same compound was designated differently in different laboratories. To eliminate this source of confusion, we use the mass of the steroid fragment as part of the common name. Note that all molecules containing only carbon, hydrogen, and oxygen atoms must have chemical formulas with an 'even" total mass number. Both nitrogen and phosphorus generate 'odd' masses except when an even number of them are present in the molecule (1+1=2). Thus, if the mass is an odd number, we know the ion is a fragment.

Phosphocholine esters will be designated as Cxxx; phosphoethanolamine esters will be designated as Exxx; Pxxx will be reserved to designate compounds for which the steroid fragment was observed but the conjugate was not confirmed by mass spectroscopy. For each symbol, the xxx will be the m/z from the steroid fragment as observed on mass spectroscopy in the cation mode. In most cases, the mass for the chemical formula of the steroid will be m/z= xxx +17 Da because the phosphoester fragment (m/z=184 Da) includes all four of the phosphate oxygen atoms, including the 3β-hydroxyl that was taken from the steroid. For steroids with carboxyl groups, the mass for the chemical formula is m/z=xxx+15 Da because carboxyl fragments must be protonated to generate a cation.

2.4. Isolation of Spiral Steroids

Rather than starting with cross reaction to an antibody to a cardiotonic steroid, our path to discovery was dependent on two physiological starting points.

First, we were investigating serum from newborn infants with Smith-Lemli-Opitz syndrome (SLO) [9]. We noted that our patient with SLO syndrome was potassium wasting. Although several diseases with sodium wasting are known, potassium wasting in newborns was not well described. Serum from our patient had high levels of unknown materials that cross-reacted with antibodies to androgen sulfates. Chromatography indicated there were two compounds present. Normal infants of the same age had 4 unidentified peaks [10]. However, none of the compounds were detectable in serum from infants after two weeks of age. Consequently, it was not possible to collect enough serum for characterization of the compounds.

Second, Bradlow had noted that fluids from human breast cysts could be characterized by their electrolyte composition [11]. Type 1 fluids had high potassium and low sodium levels while Type 2 fluids had the reverse. Together, we speculated that, to account for the difference in electrolytes, Type 1 fluids should have a compound that caused K+ accumulation and that compound might be absent in patients with SLO syndrome. From co-operating physicians, Bradlow obtained samples of both types of breast fluid. Chasalow extracted them with the methods used with the serum from newborn infants. The Type 1 fluids were very rich in the compounds that the infants with SLO didn't make [12]. This recognition provided a pathway to isolation that was distinctly different from methods suitable for isolation of digoxin or ouabain.

2.4.1. Extraction

The clinical assay for digoxin was first used to measure digoxin in patients prior to initiation of digoxin therapy [2]. The original sensitivity was 0.20 ng/ml. We modified the method to improve the sensitivity to 0.05 ng/ml. When Hamlyn had extracted normal plasma, he could not evaluate the success of his extraction method, possibly because normal levels of DLM were undetectable with the original method. In contrast, many of the Type 1 breast cyst fluid samples had levels in excess of 1.0 ng/ml with our method and even the value in the Type 1 fluid pool was 0.6 ng/ml. We tried the published extraction methods for digoxin and ouabain without success.

We identified several solvents that recovered DLM present in Type 1 (high K+) breast cyst fluids. Extraction with acetonitrile recovered most of the DLM present in the breast cyst fluids and this has been our method of choice [13].

2.4.2. Isolation from Human Breast Cyst Fluids

Our first source for successful isolation was human breast cyst fluids. On HPLC, there was one peak of DLM which had multiple, unresolved, components. One of the components had absorption at 240 nm and others did not. Repeated chromatography confirmed two major peaks were present. Component A had UV absorption over 240 nm, consistent with conjugated alkenes, but it was not a DLM. Component B did not have UV absorption over 240 nm indicating it does not have a conjugated double bond, but it was a DLM [13].

2.4.3. Isolation from Bovine and Porcine Serum

The second source was 10 L of porcine serum which we obtained from a local abattoir. We added a mass spectrometer as a supplementary HPLC detector. Component A had m/z= 496 Da (C313) and component B had m/z= 524 Da (C341). Later, we recognized that component B also contained two other components at lower concentration, one with m/z= 520 Da (C337) and the other at m/z= 522 Da (C339).

Figure 1 shows the LC-MS analysis of purified C341 obtained from porcine serum. Based on (a) the symmetrical peak shape and (b) the absence of other ions, it seems to be essentially homogeneous.

The fragmentation pattern, mass spectrum and typical amount isolated for each compound are tabulated in Table 1. The M-183 ion peak was attributed to the phosphocholine fragment and was observed with other phospholipids. The difference between the base peak at m/z=184 Da and the H+ mass ion was attributed to the steroid fragment. Thus, for the compound with m/z=496 Da, the steroid fragment would have m/z=313 Da and a fragment at that mass was present in the spectrum. The symbol for this compound would be C313. When the mass of the 3-hydroxyl group (17 Da) was added, C313 would have m/z=330 Da for the intact steroid molecule (S) and C341 would have m/z=358 of its intact molecule. However, these mass ions did not match with any known compounds.

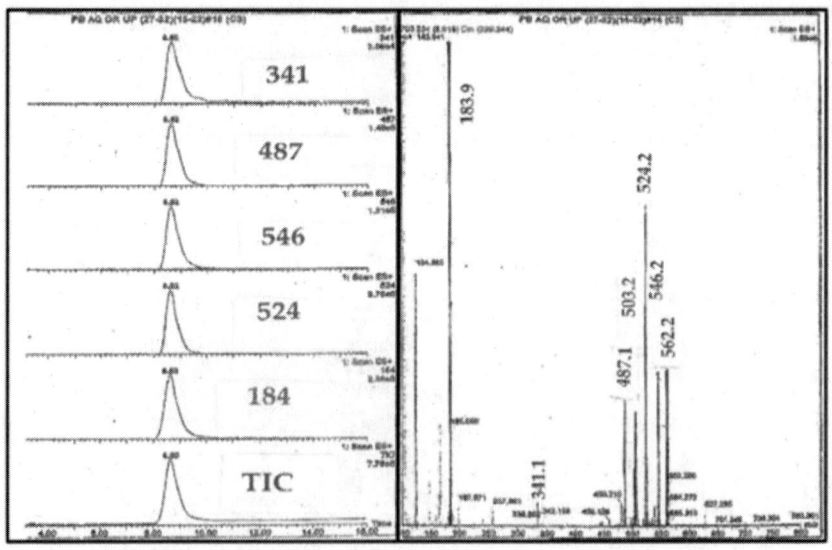

Figure 1. LC-MS analysis of m/z=524 Da (C341) from porcine serum. Left panel: Chromatograms - m/z = 341 Da; 487 Da; 546 Da; 524 Da; 184 Da; Total Ion Count (TIC). Right panel: Mass spectrum obtained at the peak of the m/z=524 Da (C341) chromatogram. Data from [8].

Table 1. Each line shows the ions and fragments of a phosphocholine ester isolated from porcine serum. Similar spectra were obtained from purified samples (estimated at >90%) from porcine serum for C313, C337 and C339. Later, with improved methods, we purified all four compounds from human and bovine serum

\multicolumn{7}{c}{Mass spectra peaks of phosphocholine esters isolated from 10 liters of porcine serum}
Symbol	Mass	M+1 Da	M+23 Da	M+23-59 Da	M-183	S
C313	20 mg	496	518	459	313	330
C337	5 mg	520	542	483	337	354
C339	5 mg	522	544	485	339	356
C341	10 mg	524	546	487	341	358

2.4.4. Model Compound: DHEA-Phosphocholine Ester

To confirm the identity of the m/z=184 Da fragment, DHEA-phosphocholine ester was synthesized from authentic DHEA [14]. A comparison of Figure 2 with Figure 1 shows the characteristic phosphocholine ion fragment at m/z=184 Da. The steroid fragment from DHEA should be m/z=271 Da. The H+ mass ion should be m/z=454 Da (271+183 = 454 Da). The Na+ ion should be at 476 Da (271+183+22 Da) and the K+ ion should be at 492 Da (271+183+39 Da). Thus, the spectrum fragmentation pattern is similar to the isolated phosphocholine steroid esters.

As a side note, we carefully searched many mass spectra for evidence of a mass ion at m/z=454 Da. We found no evidence for DHEA-phosphocholine ester in any mammalian serum or extract.

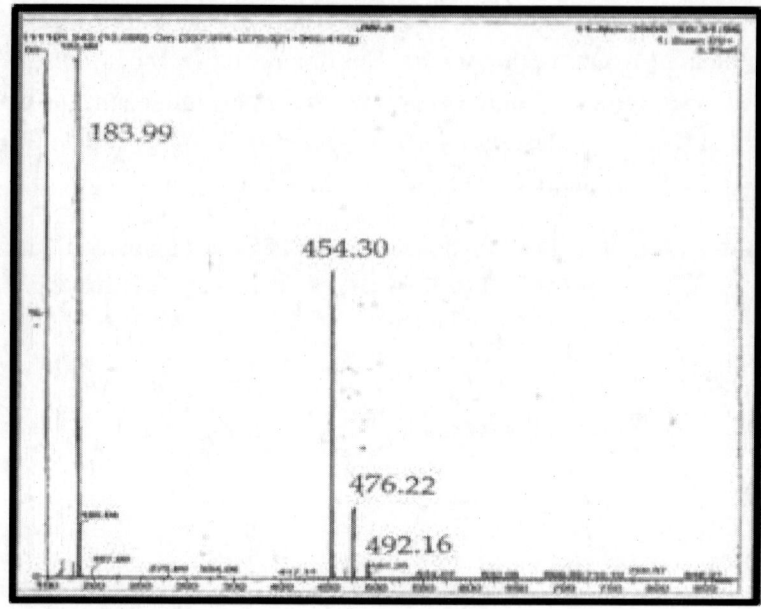

Figure 2. Mass spectrum of synthetic DHEA-phosphocholine ester.

2.5. NMR Analysis of the Steroids with 23 Carbon Atoms

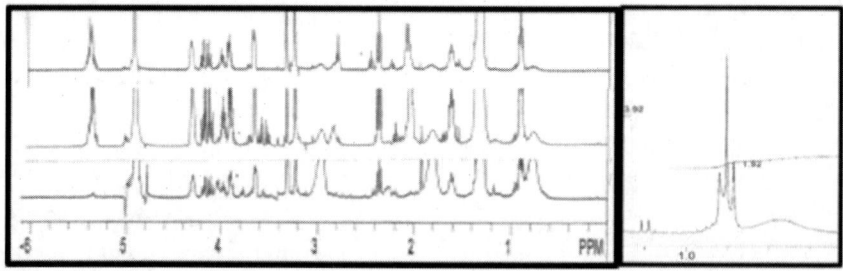

Figure 3. H-NMR analysis of spiral lactones with 23 carbon atoms [8] Left panel: Top: C337; Middle: C339; Bottom: C341 Right panel: Unsplit methyl groups are at PPM < 1.

^{1}H-NMR spectrum is shown in Figure 3. The spectrum is typical of steroids and with many different types of splitting patterns. Two features were identifiable. First, there were no long chain alkyl groups, such as a fatty acid or fatty alcohol. Second, in the panel on the side, there were three "unsplit" methyl groups. Two of these could be assigned to the angular methyl groups at carbon 18 and carbon 19. The third one is consistent with the methyl group at carbon 21, which would be unsplit, because the adjacent carbon could be either a ketone or an alkene.

2.5.1. ^{31}P-NMR Analysis of the Steroids with 23 Carbon Atoms

The ^{31}P-NMR spectra in Figure 4 confirms the molecule has one phosphorus atom. The three peaks are caused by the three cation forms – H+, Na+ and K+. ^{31}P-NMR chemical shifts vary up to several hundred, depending on the oxidation state of the phosphorus atom, confirming that these two molecules have phosphorus in a similar oxidation state.

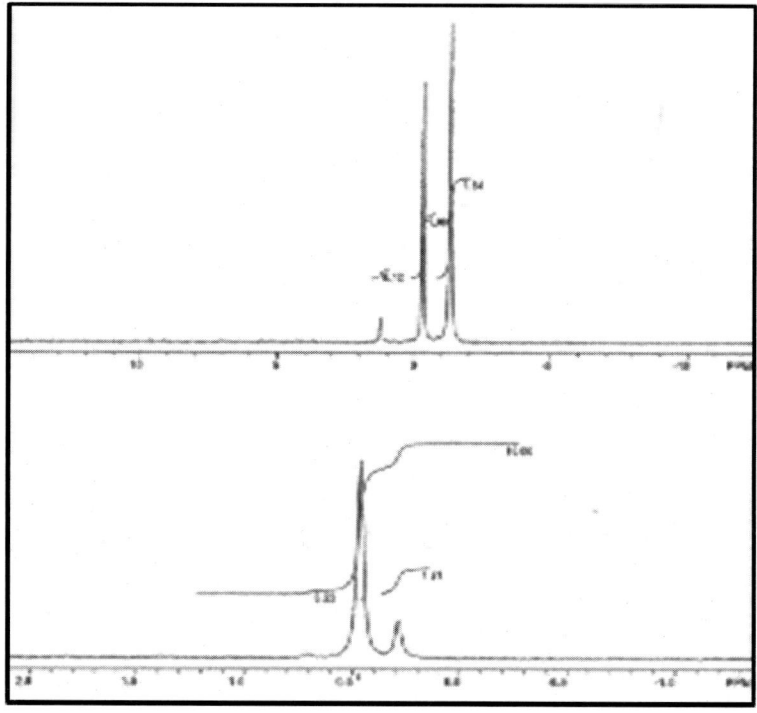

Figure 4. ^{31}P-NMR spectra of phosphocholine esters [8].
Top: ^{31}P-NMR of DHEA-PC; Bottom: ^{31}P-NMR of C341.

2.5.2. ^{13}C NMR Analysis of the Steroids with 23 Carbon Atoms

^{13}C-NMR analysis (not shown) provided a limited amount of new data. It was not consistent with a long chain alkyl group, thus eliminating structures phospholipids and platelet activating factor.

2.6. Trial-and-Error Determination of Composition

We used a trial-and-error method to evaluate possible molecular compositions for C313 and C341 (Tables 2 & 3). In the tables, after the line number, there are 6 columns. The 1st column identifies the number of carbon atoms in the trial and matches it with a number of oxygen atoms in the 2nd column. The 3rd column then calculates the contribution of the carbon and oxygen atoms to the molecular mass. The 4th column, Hreq, is the number of hydrogen atoms required to reach the desired molecular mass. Hmax is twice the number of carbon atoms plus two. Hreq can't be larger than Hmax. Delta must account for the difference between Hreq and Hmax. Each Delta reduces the need for hydrogen atoms by two. Delta includes rings and double bonds of one type or another. For a steroid-like molecule, Delta must range from 4 to 12.

This method of analysis was used to identify a likely composition for every ion fragment observed in a mass spectrum. Tables 2 and 3 are two examples.

2.6.1. Composition of C313

Table 2 shows a trial-and-error analysis of possible chemical formulas containing only carbon, oxygen and hydrogen atoms with m/z = 330 Da. Line 2 (*RED*) shows that only the chemical formula - $C_{21}H_{30}O_3$ - can make a steroid-like molecule and it must have a Delta of 7. The proposed structure (Figure 5) has: 4 Delta for the steroid rings, 2 for the alkenes at C5-6 and C7-8 and one for the ketone at C20. There may be other isomers of C313, but the composition must be $C_{21}H_{30}O_3$ with a Delta of 7.

Table 2. Molecular composition of a steroid with mass of 330 Da

Line	# of C	# of O	C+O	Hreq	Hmax	Delta
1	21	2	284	46	44	-1
2	*21*	*3*	*300*	*30*	*44*	*7*
3	21	4	316	14	44	15
4	22	3	312	18	46	14
5	23	3	324	6	48	21

2.6.2. Composition of C341 (Ionotropin)

Table 3. Trial-and-error analysis for possible compositions of molecules with a mass 358 Da (C341). The line in *RED* shows the only combination that can make a steroid-like molecule - $C_{23}H_{34}O_3$. The proposed structure (Figure 6) would have a Delta of 7: [1] 4 for the steroid ring, [2] one for E-ring, [3] one for the alkene in the E-ring and [4] one for the carboxyl group in the E-ring

Line	# of C	# of O	C + O	Hreq	Hmax	Delta
1	21	4	316	42	44	1
2	21	5	332	26	44	9
3	21	6	348	10	44	17
4	22	3	312	46	36	0
5	*23*	*3*	*324*	*34*	*48*	*7*
6	23	4	340	18	48	15
7	24	2	320	38	50	6
8	24	3	336	22	50	14

The trial-and-error analysis indicates that C341 must have 23 carbon atoms. The proposed stereochemistry is: 3β-hydroxy and 17α-hydroxy. The Δ5-6 alkene can only be directly reduced to the 5β-configuration, just like bile acids. In contrast, direct reduction of Δ4-3 ketones leads to 5α-stereochemistry. For example, reduction of testosterone leads to 5α-dihydrotestosterone.

The proposed stereochemistry is based on the stereochemistry of known enzymes catalyzing similar reactions. Even if our proposed stereochemistry is not completely correct, it does not change two facts: first – the presence of the phosphoesters was confirmed by ^{31}P-NMR analysis and, second, mass spectroscopy was used to characterize each component.

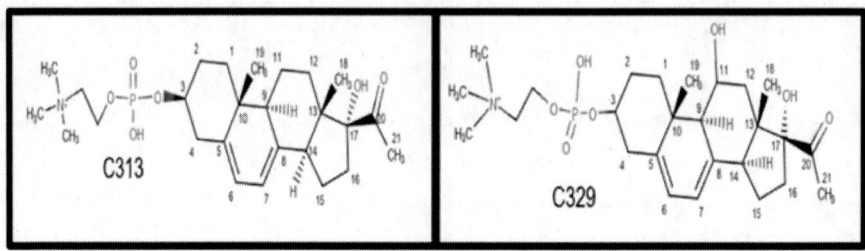

Figure 5. Family of phosphoesters with 21 carbon atoms.

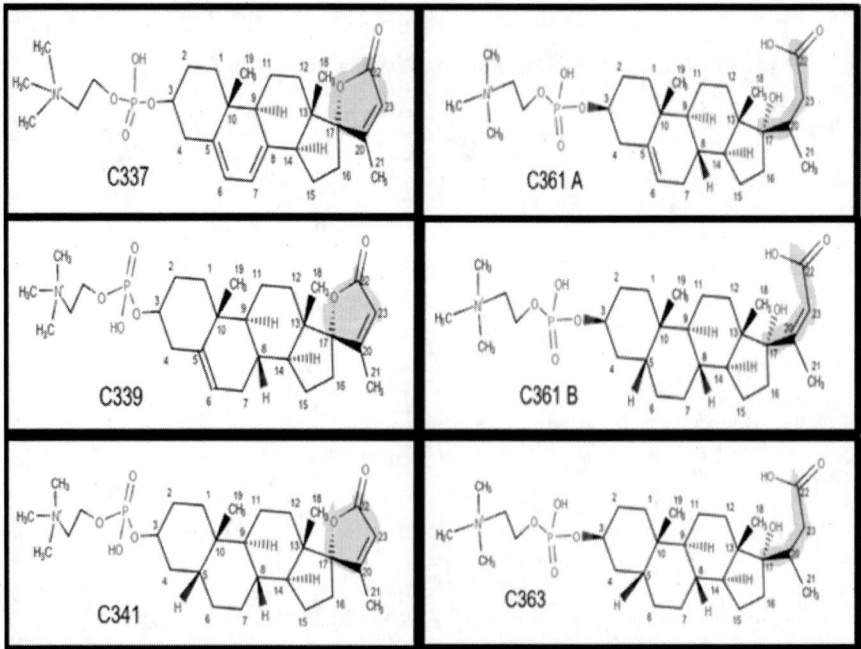

Figure 6. Family of phosphosteroids with 23 carbon atoms.

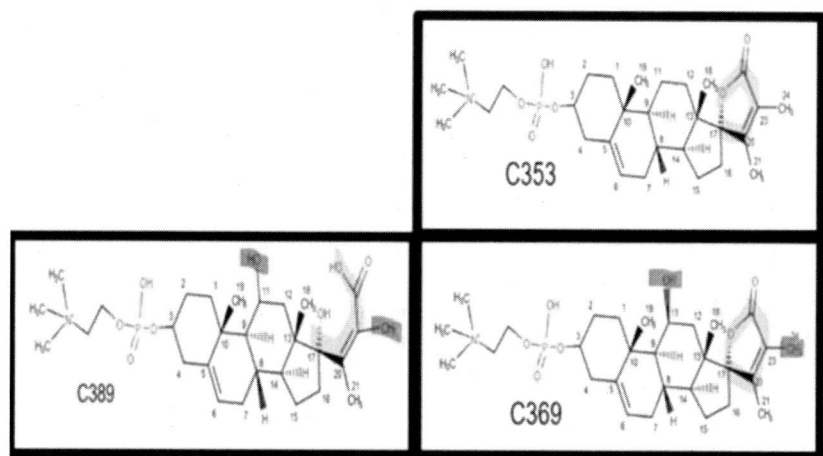

Figure 7. Family of steroids with 24 carbon atoms.

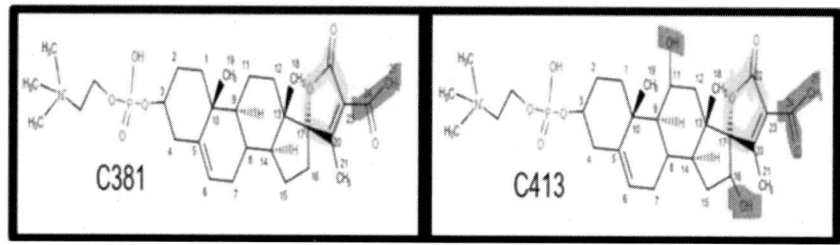

Figure 8. Family of steroids with 25 carbon atoms.

Table 4. Families and symbols of the phosphoester steroids

21 Carbon Family - C299, C313, C329!
23 Carbon Family - C337, C339, C341, C359*, C361*, C363*
24 Carbon Family - C353, C369! C389!*
25 Carbon Family - C381, C401*, P413
Proposed structural features:
  [*] E-ring not closed; [!] 11β-hydroxy-steroid.

Figures 5, 6, 7, and 8 show the proposed structures for all of the phosphoesters we have identified in mass spectra from mammals. The yellow ink shows the added carbons and the spiral lactones. Green ink is on the other components that distinguish the individual compounds. For each one, a trial-and-error analysis confirmed the molecular compositions.

The pattern indicates there are several other compounds that could exist but which we have not yet discovered. There was a fragmentation pattern for C299, but its structure is unclear.

2.6.3. Biosynthesis of Spiral Steroids

There are two ways to synthesize a steroid with 23 carbon atoms: either by [a] adding two carbon atoms to a 21-carbon atom precursor or by [b] removing four carbon atoms from a sterol, such as cholesterol. Starting with side chain labeled cholesterol, Burstein found no evidence for a four-carbon atom fragment [15] and we have not observed any ion consistent with cholesterol phosphocholine ester in any LC-MS chromatogram or MS-MS spectrum. Further, two of the isolated compounds, C313 and C337, have UV absorption characteristic of conjugated double bonds. Cholesterol can't be a precursor of C313 because cholesterol does not have a UV absorption band like C313. This suggestion is confirmed by the scarcity of successful reports of the use of cholesterol tracer to isolate a DLM and then to crystallize the product to constant specific activity. Thus, steroid phosphoesters do not derive from cholesterol.

Although cholesterol, itself, is not a precursor, this does not eliminate other sterols as possible precursors. In fact, Slominski showed that the side chain cleavage enzyme cleaved 7-dehydro-cholesterol to 7-dehydro-pregnenolone [16]. His team also isolated its 17α-hydroxy metabolite [17], which we would designate P313, if it were phosphorylated. This provides a possible steroid precursor with 21 carbon atoms for the phosphoester steroids.

Our first suggestion for the source of extra carbons was that two carbons could be added by condensation with malonyl Co-Enzyme A and subsequent decarboxylation [8]. However, that path isn't consistent with structures proposed for the families with 24 (C353) or 25 (C381) carbon atoms (Figures 7 & 8). Figure 9 shows our current proposed path. Structures B and C would probably be enzyme-bound intermediates and might not be detectable in a solvent extract. In addition to the loss of water that occurs with formation of the E-ring, the D ion would have to be protonated for it to be detected as a positive ion. Thus, D and E should be different by 20 Da, which explains the actual observation [18]. Steroid analogs to both D and E were detected for phosphoester families with 23, 24, and 25 carbon atoms.

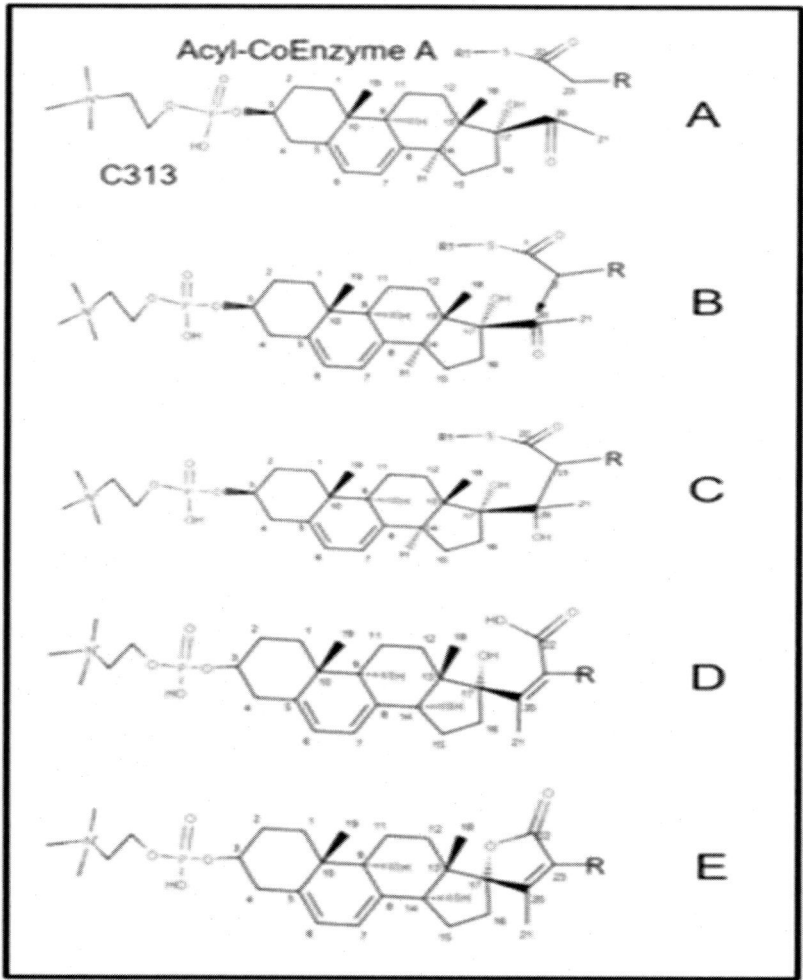

Figure 9. Proposed biosynthetic pathway to the spiral steroids.
These five structures show the steps leading to addition of 2, 3, or 4, carbon atoms to the precursor with 21-carbon atoms. The steps in the pathway are analogous to formation of long chain fatty acids.

Table 5. The CoEnzyme A acyl groups used to synthesize the families of steroids phosphoesters. There are the three most common CoEnzyme A acyl esters in mammals

R	Family	Source of carbon atoms
H	23 Carbon	Acetyl-CoEnzyme A
CH_3	24 Carbon	Propyl-CoEnzyme A
$CO-CH_3$	25 Carbon	Acetoacetyl-CoEnzyme A

2.6.4. Formation of Phosphoesters

There are two basic mechanisms for formation of Cxxx: [a] transfer of phosphocholine from another phospholipid to a steroid or [b] methylation of Exxx. However, both choline and ethanolamine are dietary requirements in mammals [19], suggesting that condensation of a steroid phosphate with either ethanolamine or choline doesn't occur in mammals. Exxx steroids are present in only trace amounts in serum. However, large amounts are present in adrenal and ovarian extracts, which are the usual sites of steroid synthesis in mammals. Although there is no specific need for the Δ7-8 alkene in the reaction, it seems to be necessary for the condensation with CDP-ethanolamine.

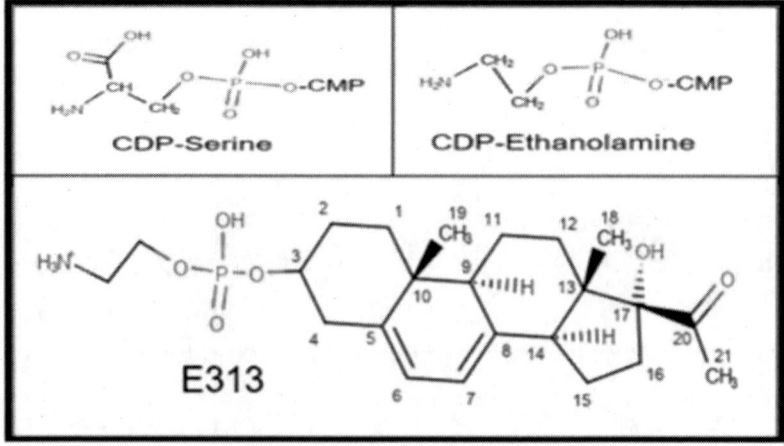

Figure 10. Synthesis of E313 from CDP-serine and a steroid.

Starting with CDP-Serine, Figure 10 shows a possible two-step pathway for the synthesis of E313. Our assumption is that E313 is the precursor for all other steroid phosphoesters. This would be consistent with accumulation of 7-dehydrosteroids [20] and hypokalemia in patients with 7-hydrosterol reductase deficiency (SLO syndrome) [10]. Exxx compounds could be storage forms, to be secreted after N-methylation.

E313 is a substrate for four different sub-pathways:

- N-methylation to C313:
  N-methylation is a B12-ACTH-dependent enzyme. It has long been known that B12 has a key role for pregnant women, but the specific process was unknown. Exxx can be stored and N-methylated to Cxxx when its specific function is needed. C313 might be metabolized to spiral steroids in tissues which do not have the enzymes for synthesis of E313.
- 11β-hydroxylation to E329:
  The ions at m/z=475 Da and at 534 Da are phosphocholine esters of E329. The proposed structure for C369, a spiral steroid with 24 carbon atoms, also includes an 11β-hydroxy component. There are two steps for synthesis of C369 from C313: 11β-hydroxylation and condensation with propyl-Co-Enzyme-A. Both intermediates (C353 and C329) are present, but the dominant path is unclear. Based on their presence in ovary and serum from pregnant women, C369 may have a role in the reproductive process [21].
- Condensation with a Co-Enzyme A acyl group:
  This enzyme leads to the three families of spiral steroids: (a) Ionotropin (C341), a 23-carbon spiral steroid which functions as a K+ sparing hormone; (b) C369, a 24-carbon spiral steroid with a role in reproduction; and (c) C381, a spiral steroid with 25 carbon atoms which is present in milk and might be responsible for high K+ levels.
- Open ring phosphoesters:
  There are several phosphoesters that are best explained as open-ring precursors for the corresponding spiral steroid lactones: C401

for C381; C389 for C369; C359 for C339; and C361 for C341. However, there is no similar match for C363. There is only one possible site for the extra two hydrogens – the C20-C23 alkene. If that is correct, then C361 may also be reduced at the C-20-C23 alkene. Potentially, one of these compounds, C361 or C363, might be a 2nd hormone in the 23-carbon atom family.

2.7. Steroid Phosphoesters in Non-Mammalian Species

Both chickens and turkeys have spiral steroids in their serum. However, both species have C339 in their serum but not C341. Chicken eggs have spiral steroids in their 'white' but not in their 'yolk' [22].

As an example of invertebrates, 'shucked' oysters were purchased at a local supermarket. The tissue was homogenized, extracted and analyzed by MS-MS [23]. Representatives of the same four families of steroid phosphoesters were identified: 21 carbon atoms, 23 carbon atoms, 24 carbon atoms and 25 carbon atoms. At least two spiral lactones, C339 and C365, were present. Our conclusion was steroid phosphoesters are not unique to mammals or even vertebrates.

2.8. Summary

There has been extended conflict about the identity of the endogenous cardiotonic glycoside or even if there is one. Other than digoxin, endogenous ouabain was the first candidate and has been extensively investigated. Since the initial claim for the discovery of endogenous ouabain in 1991 [4], there have been hundreds of papers describing (a) its pharmacology, (b) its administration in animal models and (c) its 'measurement' by radioimmunoassay in human disease [24]. One investigator has proposed its use as a less toxic substitute for digoxin in treatment of congestive heart failure [25]. Another leader in the endeavor has wondered why endogenous ouabain is not more widely accepted as the mammalian cardiotonic steroid [26]. Others have claimed endogenous ouabain is fantasy [27]. The data does not eliminate the possibility that trace amounts of endogenous ouabain, or similar compounds, might exist in mammals. What is known is that endogenous mammalian steroid phosphoesters are real. Anyone with an interest can duplicate our MS-MS experiments and document the presence of steroid phosphoesters in small volumes of mammalian serum, particularly from fetal cord serum. Their existence is not fantasy.

Whether or not mammalian cardiotonic glycosides exist [27], phosphocholine steroid esters can be isolated from mammalian tissues and sera and some of the phosphoesters are DLM. These observations differ from claims for endogenous ouabain as a mammalian DLM: (1) no potential precursors or metabolites have been identified for ouabain in mammals, (2) enzymes that could synthesize ouabain have not been identified in mammals, (3) the stereochemistry of ouabain differs from that of the usual mammalian steroids (5α vs. 5β; 14α vs. 14β) and (4) ouabain is toxic at the levels consistent with the amount claimed to have been isolated from mammalian serum.

3. FUNCTION OF SPIRAL STEROIDS (IONOTROPIN)

3.1. Background

Imagine you were a scientist in 1925 and individual steroids had not yet been identified. Imagine you had a mass spectrometer. In the laboratory, you could make an extract and analyze it with a (undiscovered) mass spectrometer. The 1925-scientist would find steroids with 18, 19, and 21 carbon atoms but wouldn't know the function of each one. We now know that the steroids with 18 carbon atoms are estrogens; the compounds with 19 carbon atoms are androgens; the compounds with 21 carbon atoms have multiple functions – progestogens, glucocorticoids and mineralocorticoids. It has taken 70 years of effort to identify the function of each compound.

I am a scientist of the 21st century. I have a mass spectrometer and have used it to characterize steroid phosphoesters. In summary, the 2020-scientist team has identified 3 different families of phosphoester steroids characterized by the number of carbon atoms, either 23, 24 or 25 carbon atoms. Although each of the families has a spiral steroid member, it does not imply that each of the spiral steroids has an identical function. There may be different receptors in different tissues. There is more to learn.

3.2. Why Do We Need Potassium Sparing Hormones?

Life started in the ocean with NaCl as the major electrolyte. Hence, a Na+ channel would be sufficient to accumulate Na+, but a pump would be needed to accumulate intracellular K+. One way of determining if a strange object is/was alive could be to determine if it was capable of maintaining an internal electrolyte composition different from its local environment.

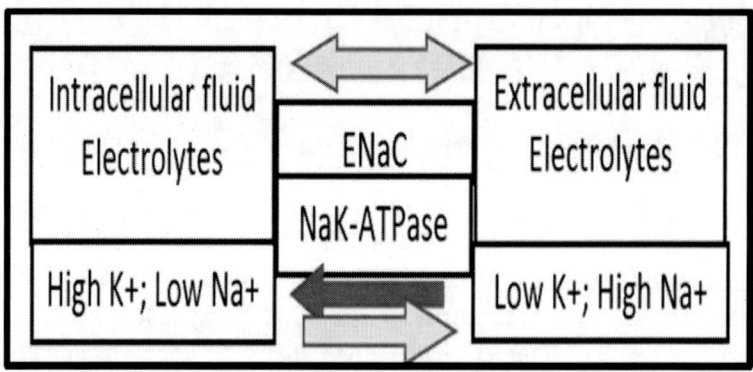

Figure 11. A simple drawing of electrolyte regulatory processes.

In most mammals, plasma electrolytes match that of sea water - 145 mM Na+ and 4-6 mM K+. In contrast, electrolytes in intracellular fluids are about 100 mM K+ and about 10 mM Na+. Passive diffusion would lead to a gain of intracellular Na+ and loss of intracellular K+. To maintain the proper electrolyte pattern, there must be an energy-requiring, transport mechanism and a regulatory mechanism.

Figure 11 shows the two key processes. The yellow arrows show the movement of Na+ ions and the blue arrow shows the movement of K+ ions. Epithelial Sodium Channels (ENaC) enhance passive diffusion of Na+ ions. As the concentration is higher in the plasma, this generally leads to Na+ entry into cells. In the kidney, ENaC recovers Na+ before it gets secreted in the nascent urine. ENaC synthesis is stimulated by mineralocorticoids, such as aldosterone. In contrast, in tissues, the NaK-ATPase requires ATP to transport K+ into cells against the gradient. In the kidney, it recovers K+ from the nascent urine. However, in contrast to Na+ recovery, no regulatory hormones were known for K+ recovery.

It is hard for a land mammal to develop hypokalemia because the level of K+ in the diet is about 40 mM and the plasma level of K+ is about 4-6 mM. Thus, passive diffusion readily recovers K+ from the diet. However, the level of K+ level in plasma is much lower than the intracellular level (60-100 mM) and wouldn't be maintained by passive diffusion. This is the function of the NaK-ATPase.

The next three sections present the evidence that Ionotropin is an endogenous potassium sparing hormone: (1) Ionotropin shares structural features with cardiotonic steroids and synthetic potassium sparing hormones; (2) Patients with SLO have symptoms consistent with hypokalemia and the defect in SLO prevents synthesis of Ionotropin; and (3) High potassium, human breast cyst fluids contain high levels of a DLM that is a spiral steroid phosphocholine ester.

3.3. Structural Features of Potassium Sparing Diuretics

There are two types of synthetic K+ sparing diuretics and they function by different mechanisms.

First, both amiloride and triamterene prevent function of Epithelial Sodium Channels (ENaC). These drugs reduce the diffusion of Na+ into cells.

Second, both spironolactone and digoxin stimulate Na-K-ATPase to transport K+ into cells and simultaneously transport Na+ out of the cells.

All of these compounds have a Ring E lactone. However, it should be noted that, in laboratory assays, spironolactone and digoxin inhibit the NaK-ATPase. If that were the case *in vivo*, it could not restore intracellular K+ concentration. There is no other known mechanism to maintain intracellular K+ levels to compensate for gradient-independent K+ diffusion. Thus, a major paradigm shift is needed to account for intracellular electrolyte regulation. There are two parts to the new paradigm: (1) the discovery of spiral steroids, including Ionotropin and (2) spiral steroid regulation of NaK-ATPase.

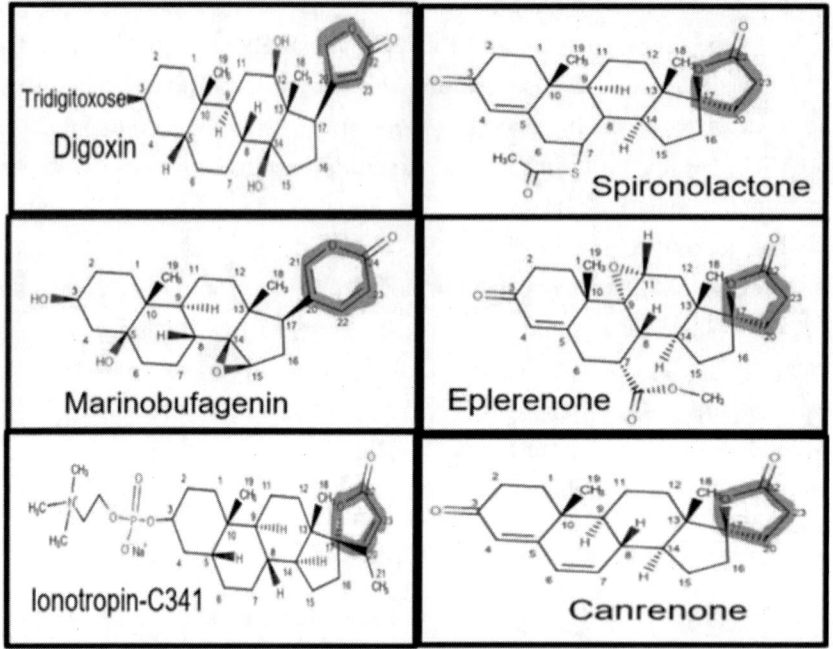

Figure 12. Structures of some K+ sparing drugs and hormones. The lactone E-ring is highlighted in green.

Figure 12 shows six compounds that function as K+ sparing diuretics. The left-hand column shows three natural compounds. Digoxin was originally isolated from *digitalis lanata*. Marinobufagenin was isolated from toad skin [28]. Ionotropin was isolated from cattle, pigs and humans [8]. The right-hand column shows three synthetic diuretics. Immunoassays, using digoxin specific antibodies, detect all six compounds. Although there are claims for isolation of digoxin, ouabain and marinobufagenin from mammalian plasma and tissue, no intermediates or metabolites have been identified. For Ionotropin, we have identified precursor and metabolites and we isolated mg amounts of 6 different phosphocholine steroid esters. In summary, all six of the compounds shown in the figure are DLM and all six of these compounds inhibit NaK-ATPase when measured in the laboratory. On that basis, we propose that Ionotropin functions as a potassium sparing hormone.

3.4. Do Spiral Steroids Have Nuclear Receptors?

When we isolated Ionotropin (C341) from 10 liters of porcine blood, the final product weighed about 10 mg (see Table 1) [8]. This corresponds to an original concentration of 1000 µg/L or about 2 µM. For comparison, (1) normal adult males have a testosterone level of 300 ng/dl or 1 nmol/dl or ~10 nM; (2) normal adult standing levels of aldosterone are 7-30 ng/dl or <1 nM. These numbers indicate that a spiral steroid nuclear receptor, similar to those for testosterone or aldosterone, would be saturated and internalized at all times if the receptor had an affinity similar to one of those receptors.

There is only one steroid with higher serum levels than Ionotropin. It is dehydroepiandrosterone sulfate (DHEA-S). Young adult serum levels are ~300 µg/dl or ~10 µM. No nuclear receptors have been identified and no specific function for DHEA-S as a hormone has been established.

3.5. SLO Syndrome – Spiral Steroid Deficiency

The underlying pathology of SLO Syndrome is 7-dehydrosterol reductase deficiency. Patients with this syndrome accumulate 7-dehydrocholesterol [20]. Symptoms of the syndrome include hypokalemia and agenesis of the kidney and the heart. In mildly affected infants, the hypokalemia spontaneously resolves during the first week post-partum. Two events occur during the first week of life: fetal spiral lactones are metabolized and newborn nutrition is switched from low K+ plasma to milk, which is rich in K+. Thus, hypokalemia ends because renal diffusion recovers K+ without the need for a potassium sparing hormone.

This syndrome was originally recognized on the basis of morphological features, but there were also endocrine features. The three typical steroid-dependent organs, gonads, heart, and kidney were incompletely formed. Patients were potassium wasting and benefited from digoxin therapy [10]. Although not recognized at the time, this pattern defines spiral steroid deficiency and characterizes the target organs for hyper-spirolemia [21]. If potassium was inadequate, then spiral steroids would be needed and synthesized, leading to hypertension and proteinuria. Sounds like pre-eclampsia to me.

3.6. Human Breast Cyst Fluids

In the 1970s and 1980s, breast cysts were investigated as potential precursors of breast cancer. Consequently, there was extensive investigation of the hormones and processes in the cyst fluids [11]. The most striking biochemical observation was that electrolytes divided the fluids into two types. Type 1 fluids had 60-100 mM K+ levels and 10-20 mM Na+ levels. Type 2 had 5-10 mM K+ levels and 100 mM Na+ levels. The first hypothesis was that the Type 1 might be the cancer precursor and the Type 2 fluids might be benign. Investigation of 1700 cysts showed there was no association of electrolyte type with breast cancer. However, as described in Section 1.4.2, there were differences in the DLM concentration. DLM was elevated in the Type 1 fluids and was undetectable in the Type 2 fluids [12]. We proposed that the compound that the SLO syndrome patients couldn't make, might be present in the Type 1 fluids and be responsible for the accumulation of K+ in the cyst fluids against the gradient.

3.7. Summary

In brief, spiral steroids have three significant features: [a] potassium wasting occurs in their absence, [b] potassium accumulates in fluids in which it is present and [c] they share specific structural features with the steroid class of potassium sparing diuretics. In contrast to the 'evidence' for endogenous ouabain, we have identified precursors, the biosynthetic pathway and a mass spectroscopy method of assay suitable for use on individual serum samples.

4. PHOSPHOSTEROIDS DURING PREGNANCY

4.1. Background

During pregnancy, there are two key sites of potassium nutrition: the maternal compartment and the fetal compartment. When maternal kidneys are functioning normally, the amount of potassium in the diet is more than sufficient.

The fetus is in a different circumstance. Potassium is needed for two functions: first, to maintain intracellular potassium levels and second, as the fetus grows, for an inotropic affect to maintain cardiovascular perfusion. These requirements reach a maximum about halfway through pregnancy, coinciding with the classical symptoms of pre-eclampsia - hypertension and proteinuria. For both functions, potassium must be pumped from the fetal plasma at a low potassium concentration (~5 mM) into fetal tissues which have a much higher potassium concentration (~100 mM). Because of the natural concentration gradient, increasing blood flow does not provide a driving force to transfer potassium ions to the intracellular fluid compartment. The driving force can only be provided by activation of an ATP-dependent electrolyte transferase.

4.2. Concept: Role of Spiral Steroids

Figure 13 illustrates the changes in potassium electrolytes that occur during pregnancy. The biology has been known, but the underlying biochemistry has not been known [29]. What makes this diagram unique is its correlation of the potassium electrolytes with phosphosteroids.

At parturition, fetal spiral steroids are 10 times adult normal levels. Coincidentally with the onset of aldosterone insensitivity, the elevated levels begin during the third trimester. Our theory is that the aldosterone signaling defect is caused by spiral steroids. The aldosterone signaling defect leads to fetal sodium wasting, which is a necessary step for formation of amniotic fluid.

It is our theory the process is 'all about potassium' [30]. If potassium levels are insufficient, the mother responds by making spiral steroid precursors. The fetal-placental unit converts the precursors to spiral steroids. The spiral steroids stimulate the fetal NaK-ATPase which, in turn, pumps potassium into cells, increases blood pressure and causes sodium wasting by the fetus. If this begins to early, at 20-22 weeks of gestational age, we characterize the process as pre-eclampsia. If the response is exaggerated or mistimed, then maternal hyper-spirolemia leads to life threatening hypertension, just as would occur with an overdose of a cardiotonic glycoside. This same transport process involving steps in the maternal, fetal and placental compartments also occurs with estriol.

Ions A, B, and C were observed in every mammalian serum sample that was analyzed. The identity of each ion was confirmed by MS-MS analysis. For example, ions at m/z = 546 Da (designated C) were collected in the MS-MS trap and further fragmented. The spectrum is shown in the right-hand panel of Figure 14. The daughter ion is m/z = 487 Da, derived by loss of trimethylamine (59 Da). The 487 Da ion further fragmented to grand-daughter ions at m/z = 341 Da and 146 Da. This confirmed ion C in the fetal calf serum is the Na+ cation of C341.

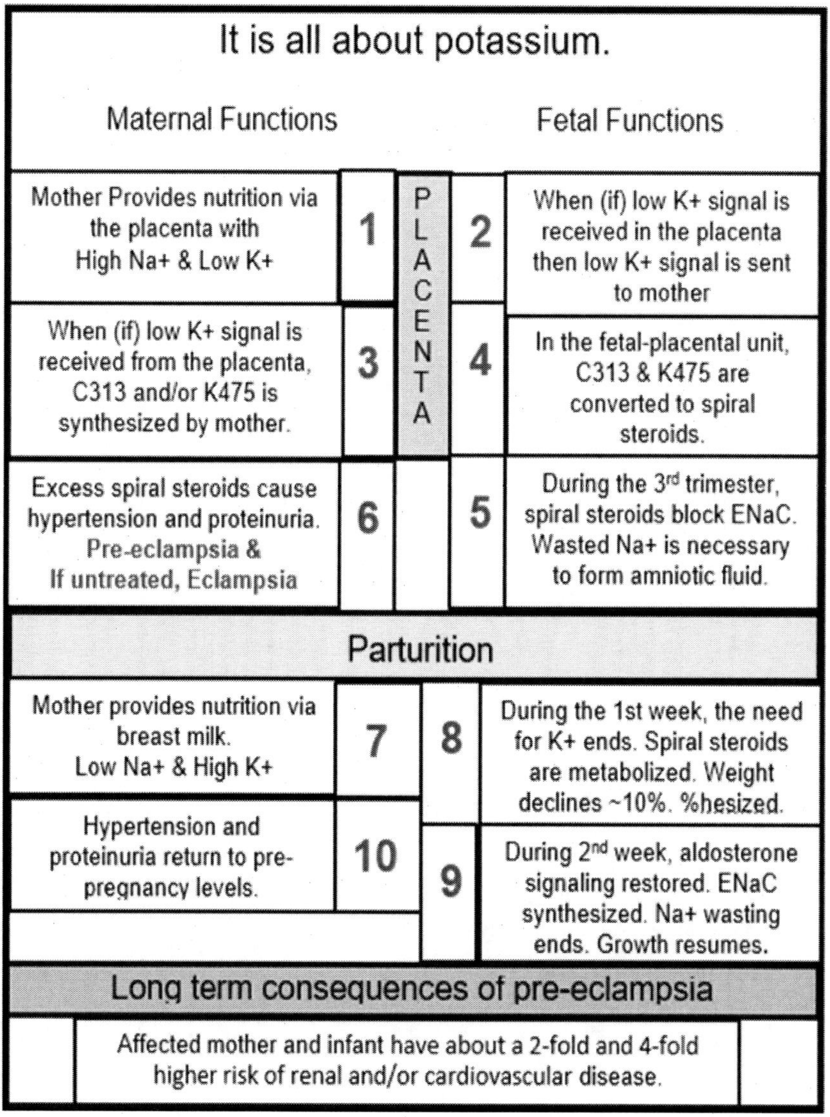

It is all about potassium.

Maternal Functions				Fetal Functions
Mother Provides nutrition via the placenta with High Na+ & Low K+	1	P L A C E N T A	2	When (if) low K+ signal is received in the placenta then low K+ signal is sent to mother
When (if) low K+ signal is received from the placenta, C313 and/or K475 is synthesized by mother.	3		4	In the fetal-placental unit, C313 & K475 are converted to spiral steroids.
Excess spiral steroids cause hypertension and proteinuria. Pre-eclampsia & If untreated, Eclampsia	6		5	During the 3rd trimester, spiral steroids block ENaC. Wasted Na+ is necessary to form amniotic fluid.

Parturition

Mother provides nutrition via breast milk. Low Na+ & High K+	7		8	During the 1st week, the need for K+ ends. Spiral steroids are metabolized. Weight declines ~10%. %hesized.
Hypertension and proteinuria return to pre-pregnancy levels.	10		9	During 2nd week, aldosterone signaling restored. ENaC synthesized. Na+ wasting ends. Growth resumes.

Long term consequences of pre-eclampsia

Affected mother and infant have about a 2-fold and 4-fold higher risk of renal and/or cardiovascular disease.

Figure 13. It's all about potassium and potassium sparing hormones.

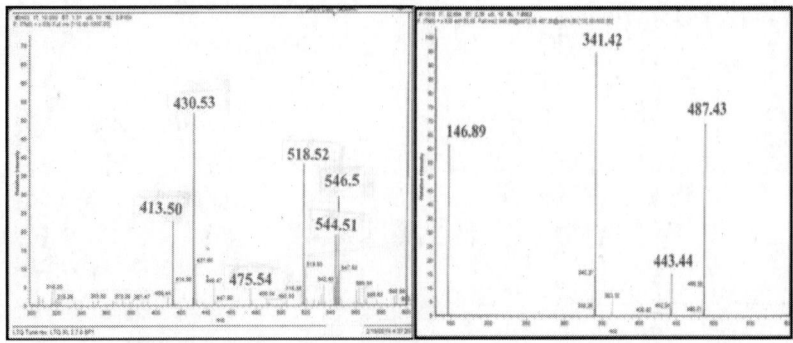

Figure 14. Mass spectra of phosphocholine steroids in fetal calf serum. Left Panel: Mass spectrum obtained by direct injection of extract from fetal calf serum. Peak A – 518 Da; Peak B – 544 Da; Peak C - 546 Da; Peak D – 413 Da; Miltefosine – 430 Da. Right Panel: MS-MS spectrum obtained by fragmentation of m/z=546 Da. This spectrum confirms that the ion at m/z=546 Da is C341 (Ionotropin).

Ion D at m/z = 413 Da has not yet been observed in any other sample from any species. The significance of the 'odd' mass of ion D is it must be generated by loss of either the phosphoethanolamine or phosphocholine fragment. Either precursor could generate a fragment with m/z= 430 Da (413 +17 Da) and be designated as P413. Ion D could not be derived from miltefosine as that compound has no hydroxy groups and could not fragment with loss of 18 Da.

Trial and error analysis of ion D suggested a composition of $C_{25}O_6H_{34}$ with Delta=9. This composition is consistent with di-hydroxy-C381 (Figure 8). There are a limited number of enzymes catalyzing steroid hydroxylation: 11, 16, 17, 18, & 21 are the most common. 21-Hydroxylase requires Δ4-3 ketones for the substrate. 17-Hydroxy is already part of the spiral steroid. An 18-hydroxy group would enhance mineralocorticoid function, but that is opposite the function of potassium sparing hormones. 16-Hydroxylation is required for the synthesis of estriol, which is a major estrogen during pregnancy. Thus, the two extra hydroxy groups seem to be at carbon atoms 11 and 16, as shown in Figure 8.

The low intensity ion at m/z = 475 Da is derived from m/z=534 Da (C329) by loss of the trimethylamine from the phosphocholine moiety. C329 could have a hydroxy group at either carbon 11 or 16. The common isomer is assumed to be the 11 hydroxy derivative, primarily on the basis of its presence in serum samples from both adult males and females.

In the m/z range from 300 to 600 Da, each of the major ions in the cation mass spectrum can be identified.

4.2.1. Human Cord Serum Investigations

Over the years, Chasalow collaborated on several investigations of fetal function. The only sample that can be collected without risk to the fetus is the umbilical cord sample obtained at parturition [30]. In one study we evaluated growth hormone isoforms in infants. The work scope was divided into two parts: Dr. Kathryn King oversaw the collection of samples and I oversaw the laboratory evaluation. To collect cord samples at the time of parturition, a portion of the cord was 'double' clamped and serum was collected by needle biopsy, specifically from the umbilical artery. Although the literature suggests that cord serum hCG levels are 90 ± 5 mIU/ml, our analysis of individual samples describes a different distribution. Of 173 samples assayed for hCG, only 16 had levels above 90 mIU/ml, clearly indicating a mean of 90 +5 mIU/ml is impossible.

In a second study with Dr. Sharon Nachman, we investigated 22 cord serum samples from mothers with HIV infection [31]. 7 of the 8 samples with hCG levels over 90 mIU/ml were shown to be HIV infected. Of the 14 infants with low hCG levels only 3 were HIV infected. The association was statistically significant at the p=0.02 level. Our conclusion was that there was a process that transferred both hCG and HIV from the maternal to the fetal circulation. The cause of the difference between our normal population and the previously reported data is probably the care we took in our sample collection method which avoided contamination from maternal serum and the umbilical vein.

In a third study, we evaluated DLM levels in umbilical cord samples. The average DLM was over 0.6 ng/ml, ten times more than normal adults or children. We don't know which DLM was present because we did not have access to a mass spectrometer [33].

4.2.2. Infants Postpartum

After parturition, as an infant adapts to extrauterine life, there are three stages in electrolyte metabolism [34].

In the first week, infants experience an initial oliguria followed by diuresis and natriuresis. Most infants experience a loss of about 10% of their weight. This occurs simultaneously with the change in nutrition from plasma with low potassium levels (4-7 mM) to milk with high potassium levels (60-100 mM). The weight loss and nutritional change are well known, but the underlying biochemistry was unknown. Aldosterone levels are unchanged but, initially, the third trimester signaling defect is still intact. Fetal levels of spiral steroids are maintained briefly, leading to continued salt wasting. Overall, during the first stage, the biochemistry of adaption fits with our experiments showing the presence of a potassium sparing hormone, Ionotropin, in cord serum and its disappearance from serum by the end of the first week [29].

During the second week, because milk is rich in potassium, synthesis of potassium sparing hormones are terminated; aldosterone signaling resumes; the sodium balance turns positive; weight loss ends and growth resumes [10].

After the second week, growth is characterized by continuous weight gain. The biological changes have been known. Our research has provided the biochemical underpinnings for the process.

4.3. Pre-Eclampsia - Syndrome or Disease?

At present, pre-eclampsia fits the definition of a syndrome [35]. The classical symptoms are hypertension and proteinuria as early as 20 weeks of gestational age, but the underlying pathology is unknown [36]. During the third trimester, about 5% of affected women develop life threatening hypertension [37]. After childbirth, affected women are also at long-term, increased risk of renal failure [38], high blood pressure, heart disease and stroke [39]. To date, there are no FDA approved methods for diagnosis or progression and, to encourage research, pre-eclampsia has even been designated as an orphan disease [40]. One key factor seems to be improper implantation [41]. Although improper implantation has been well documented, proximal causes for pre-eclampsia and/or life-threatening hypertension are unknown. In brief, biology is known but pathology is not. After childbirth, none of the proposed markers provide any insight into the pathogenesis of the maternal increased risk of renal or heart disease. We can't even distinguish if (a) the risk is pre-existing before pregnancy or if (b) the risk is caused by an unidentified mechanism in women who experience pre-eclampsia.

For more than 30 years, there has been a concerted effort to identify potential biomarkers for pre-eclampsia. Without going into extensive details, anything that could be measured as a potential predictive marker for pre-eclampsia, has been measured [42]. The search has concentrated on four methods [43]:

- Ultrasonic methods
- Molecular markers in the maternal circulation
- Clinical history
- First trimester blood pressure.

In 1987, Graves initiated one of the first efforts to convert pre-eclampsia from a syndrome to a disease [44]. He observed that many women with pre-eclampsia had elevated levels of an unknown material that could be detected by digoxin-specific antibodies (DLM). However, the compound and its function have remained elusive. Prior to our isolation and characterization of the spiral steroids, endogenous cardiotonic steroids could only be measured by immuno-assay based on antibodies selected for poisons isolated from plants or amphibians. What Graves detected in serum from women with pre-eclampsia remains unknown [44].

4.4. Pre-Eclampsia and Spiral Steroids

Our discovery of the spiral steroids and the recognition of their role as potassium sparing hormones opens a new approach. Fetal nutrition is provided via the placenta. Maternal plasma electrolyte concentrations are 145 mM Na+ and 5-6 mM K+ and fetal plasma electrolytes are basically similar. However, fetal tissue intracellular electrolytes are about 100 mM K+ and 60 mM Na+. Thus, Na+ could enter cells by diffusion but there should be a mechanism to concentrate K+ against the concentration gradient and that hormone might be a spiral steroid which Graves would have suggested was a DLM.

4.4.1. Pilot Study

For this study [45], we purchased 40 samples from Global Alliance for the Prevention of Prematurity and Stillbirth (GAPPS). GAPPS did not disclose any characteristics about the samples other than that the 40 samples were obtained from pregnant women of 22-24 months gestational age. Samples were double blinded, first by GAPPS and then by Dr. Bochner. When samples were received in the laboratory, the sample vials were assigned a third random code number. After the laboratory results were submitted to Dr. Bochner, GAPPS provided the diagnosis. At that time, the laboratory learned (1) there were 20 normotensive and 20 women with pre-eclampsia and (2) there were 10 male and 10 female fetuses in each group.

4.4.2. Method of Analysis

For analysis, miltefosine (hexadecyl phosphocholine) was added as an internal control. Each sample was extracted and evaluated by tandem MS. Considering that samples were prepared for analysis by a simple extract and filter procedure, the clarity of the data was amazing. The method detected all of the steroid phosphoesters, including both the spiral steroids and their precursors.

For each mass ion, the ion counts were compared to the ion counts of miltefosine. The samples from the normotensive women were used to establish the mean and standard deviation. Z-scores were then determined for each of the serum components.

4.4.3. Normotensive & Pre-Eclampsia Mass Spectra

Table 6. Ions in serum from pregnant woman

m/z (Da)	Symbol	Proposed structures
430		Miltefosine
353	P353	23-methyl-P339
381	P381	23-aceto-P339
475	C329	11β-hydroxy- C313
518	C313	
546	C341	

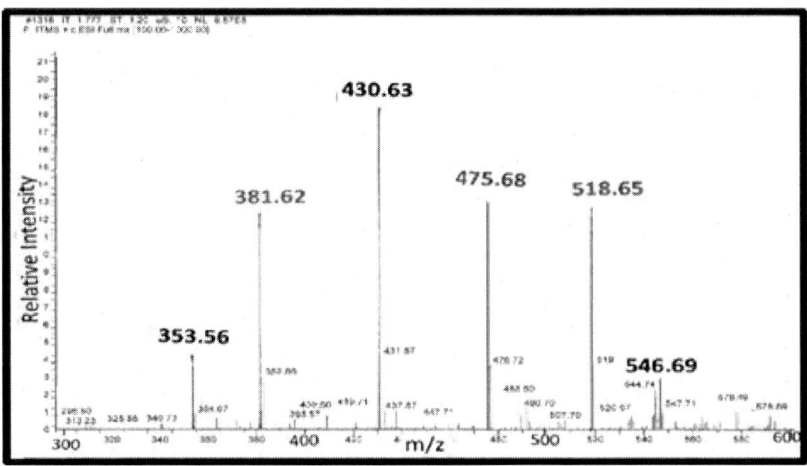

Figure 15. Mass spectrum obtained from serum of a normotensive pregnant woman [45].

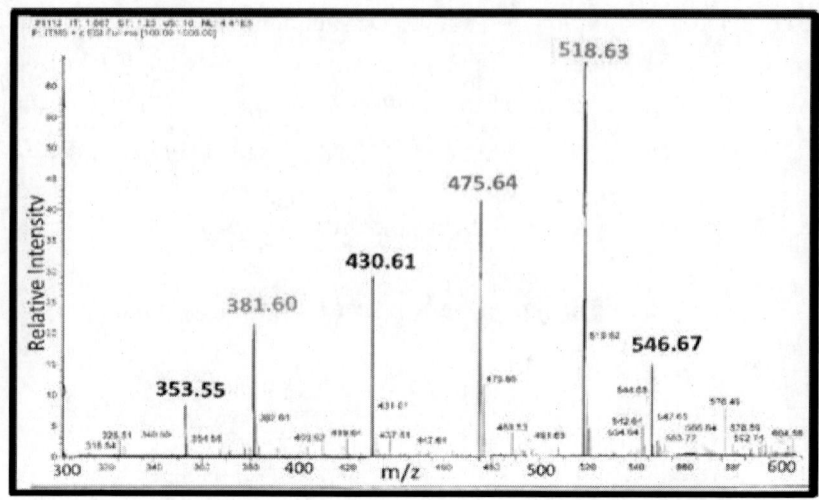

Figure 16. Mass spectrum obtained from serum of a woman with pre-eclampsia [45].

4.4.4. Identification of the Ions in Serum from Pregnant Women

- Miltefosine: The m/z observed is at m/z=430 Da. The formula mass of Miltefosine as the free acid is 408 Da. The m/z observed is at m/z=430 Da. The ion detected is the Na+ cation. The K+ cation would have a formula mass of 446 Da. This was not observed, confirming that K+ had not been added in the process of obtaining the serum samples. The low ion counts for the m/z=408 Da ion confirms that most ions were Na+ cations. This simplifies understanding of the serum components.
- Ion detected - m/z=518 Da. Assignment – Na+ cation of C313.

As shown in Figure 2, synthetic steroid phosphoesters, when analyzed by LC-MS, generate a spectrum with 5 peaks. As shown in Table 1, one of the ions derived from C313 is the Na+ ion at m/z=518 Da.

- Ion detected - m/z=475 Da. Assignment - Na+ cation after loss of trimethylamine from ion m/z= 534 Da. Steroid fragment would be m/z=329 Da. The mass ion is odd, confirming it is a fragment generated by loss of trimethylamine (59 Da). MS-MS analysis

confirmed the parent ion is 534 Da. An oxygen atom would add 16 Da to C313. The trial-and-error analysis was consistent with the extra oxygen atom. C329 was not detected in serum from pre-pubertal children of either sex (8).
- Ion detected – m/z=P381 Da. Assignment - steroid fragment: phosphoester unidentified.

P381 could be the 23-acetoacetyl derivative of C339. Figure 8 shows a possible structure. This structure is consistent with condensation of C313 with acetoacetyl- CoEnzyme A.

- Ion detected - m/z=353 Da: Assignment - P353: phosphoester unidentified. P353 could be the 23-methyl derivative of C339. It would be formed by condensation of C313 with propyl Coenzyme A, rather than acetyl Coenzyme A. P353 was first thought to be an unknown contaminant. The detection of C369 and C389 seems to confirm the assignment.
- Ion detected - m/z=546 Da: Assignment – The Na+ cation of C341 (Ionotropin).

Summary: C341, C353, and C381 are spiral steroids with 23, 24, and 25 carbon atoms. C313 and C329 are spiral steroid precursors with 21-carbon atoms.

4.4.5. Pilot Study - Z-Scores

Z-scores of the individual samples are shown in Figure 17 for normotensive women and Figure 18 for the women who were diagnosed with pre-eclampsia. At 22-24 weeks of gestation, there was no elevation in Ionotropin (C341 - m/z=546 Da), C353, or C381 in the maternal circulation of women with pre-eclampsia when compared to normotensive, pregnant women. Serum levels of spiral steroids don't show an episodic secretory pattern, such as is observed with cortisol, but that doesn't mean there is no variation of serum levels. Serum levels of spiral steroids in women with pre-eclampsia might be elevated but still be within the range defined by normotensive pregnant women.

First, we calculated the means and standard deviations of the ion intensities of C313, C329 and C381 from the control group. The individual Z-scores are shown in Figure 17. One sample had $Z > 2$. For a normal distribution, 95% of the samples should be within 2 standard deviations of the mean and about 2/3 of the samples should be within 1 standard deviation of the mean. Both of these criteria were satisfied for the control group. A positive test was defined as $Z > 2$ for one of the spiral steroid precursors, either C313 or C329.

Second, based on the data from the control group, we calculated Z-scores for C313 and C329 for the women with pre-eclampsia. The distribution of the Z-scores was not from the same population as the control group. There were too many samples with $Z > 2$ and the samples not clustered around the mean. Specifically, 11 of 19 (58%) samples had $Z > 2$ for at least one of the spiral steroid precursors. The 20th sample was not included in the analysis because it showed signs of hydrolysis. The statistical significance for this distribution of positive test result is $P < 0.001$. The distribution of Z-scores for C381 were within normal ranges.

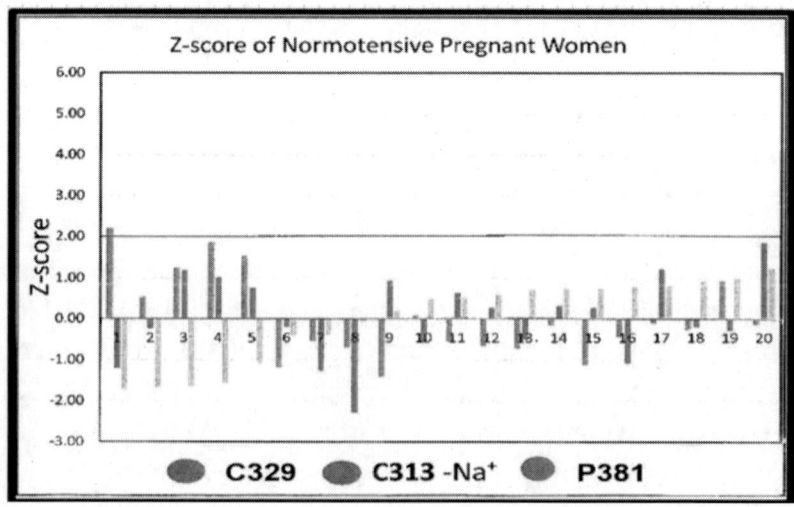

Figure 17. Z scores of phosphoesters from normotensive women.

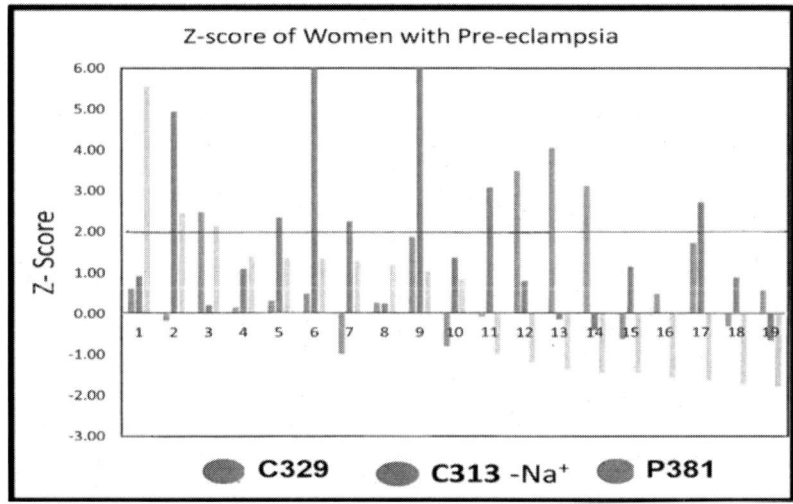

Figure 18. Z scores of women with pre-eclampsia.

4.4.6. Comparison of Elevated Precursor Levels to Other Proposed Markers for Pre-Eclampsia

Current markers under development for risk of pre-eclampsia have prediction scores of less than 40% [46]. Investigators are currently exploring multi-component tests, similar in concept to the triple test for risk of trisomy 21 [47], but, so far, these have failed to reach statistical significance [48, 49, 50].

Based on positive test symptoms at 22-24 weeks of gestation, the pilot study divides patients with pre-eclampsia into two groups: [a] a disease and [b] a syndrome 'stub'.

- Disease – hypertension, proteinuria, inadequate potassium, hyper-steroid precursors, premature synthesis of spiral steroids,
- 'Stub' – hypertension, proteinuria, without hyper-steroid precursors.

The suggestion that pre-eclampsia syndrome is not a single disease may explain the lack of development of a therapeutic approach.

With our discovery of the spiral steroids and the elevated levels of the precursors documented in some patients, we now have a basis for monitoring progression and testing therapies.

The positive test result might be the proximate cause of the classical symptoms of pre-eclampsia and might be the basis for the long-term increased incidence of renal and cardiac diseases.

The 'stub' syndrome might be a transient effect that occurs while the mother adjusts her metabolism to provide adequate potassium levels and may have no long-term consequence.

4.5. Pathophysiology of Pre-Eclampsia as a Disease

Potassium is a key nutrient for the fetus. When potassium is adequate in the fetus, it is used for [i] intracellular fluid electrolytes and, [ii] as the capillary bed expands, maintains perfusion in the periphery by improving cardiac function. During the 3rd trimester, aldosterone insensitivity causes fetal sodium wasting. This process plays an important role because the 'wasted' electrolytes form the amniotic fluid [34]. Our investigation of the fetal calf serum confirmed spiral steroids were present (Figure 14). In fact, human cord serum contains levels of spiral steroids that are 10 times higher than normal adult levels [33, 51]. The control group of the study showed that, during the mid-2nd trimester period, normotensive pregnant women do not have elevated levels of the precursors. To account for the spiral steroids in the cord serum, fetal levels of the precursors must rise during the 3rd trimester.

As illustrated in Figure 13, potassium becomes an important fetal nutrient during the 2nd trimester. Inadequate potassium levels could be caused by errors in implantation, by excessive fetal size, or by other errors in placental function. We propose that, in response to inadequate potassium levels, the mother synthesizes spiral steroid precursors. These are converted to spiral steroids in the fetal-placental compartment, function as potassium sparing hormones, and are the proximate cause of the classical symptoms of pre-eclampsia.

4.6. Summary – Spiral Steroids vs Cardiotonic Glycosides

The physiology of spiral steroids resembles the pharmacology of cardiotonic glycosides. Figure 12 compares the structure of cardiotonic glycosides to the proposed structure of a spiral steroid, C341. Both cardiotonic glycosides and C341 inhibit NaK-ATPase and both are detectable in serum from pregnant women in the 3rd trimester, when aldosterone function is blocked. Digi-bind lowers blood pressure in women with pre-eclampsia, just as it does in patients experiencing digoxin toxicity [52]. Pre-eclampsia resembles the endocrine changes that would be expected if a patient had an overdose of a cardiotonic glycoside. However, no one has confirmed the presence of a cardiotonic glycoside in serum from a patient with pre-eclampsia by any method other than by immunochemistry with antibodies to plant or amphibian cardiotonic glycosides. In contrast, we confirmed the presence of spiral steroids and their precursors by mass spectroscopy.

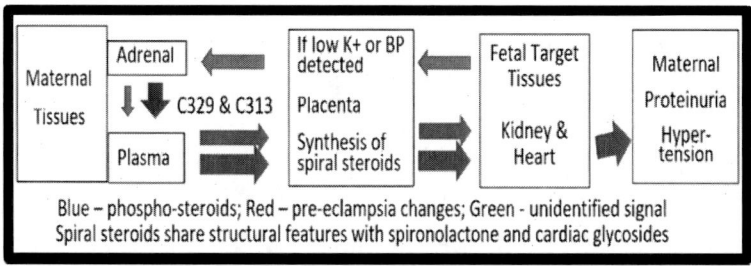

Figure 19. Proposed pathophysiology of pre-eclampsia (disease).

4.7. Proposed Clinical Application

Identification and application of a marker, like the spiral steroids and/or their precursors, C313 and C329, provides a basis for monitoring disease progression and permits development of improved therapeutic modalities. The early identification of patients needing a higher level of scrutiny during the remainder of pregnancy might result in reduced maternal/fetal morbidity and mortality.

In the pilot study, we observed that about 40% of patients have classical clinical symptoms of pre-eclampsia but no evidence of elevated levels of spiral steroids or their precursors. The basis for their pathology and its consequences has yet to be elucidated. It may be a transient effect because it is not reinforced by synthesis of spiral steroid precursors during the 2nd trimester. Women with a negative test would be pleased to know they are not in the high-risk group, if that was true.

5. PRE-ECLAMPSIA AND LIFE-THREATENING HYPERTENSION

The bottom row shows the changes in spiral steroids in normotensive, pregnant women. We already reported that cord serum has high levels of spiral steroids [33]. Thus, in order to accumulate the high levels of spiral steroids, maternal synthesis of precursors must begin in the 3rd trimester [18]. This coincides with the block in aldosterone signaling that occurs in the 3rd trimester [34] and which is necessary to form amniotic fluid. The block was known to exist but its identity was unknown.

The top row shows the proposed consequences of inadequate serum potassium levels during the 2nd trimester. The pilot study showed about 60% of patients with pre-eclampsia begin synthesis of spiral steroid precursors by 20-22 weeks of gestational age [45]. This is shown by the third circle. The fourth circle shows the early production of spiral steroids. In some women, the disorder progresses to life-threatening hypertension. In summary, pre-eclampsia seems to be a normal process occurring at an abnormal time; we propose the sequence starts with inadequate potassium levels.

There are 6 different spiral steroids (C339, C341, C353, C369, C381, and C413) that have C313 or C329 as a precursor. The pattern may predict which individuals are at increased risk of life-threatening hypertension during the 3rd trimester. There have been many studies proposing various defects in implantation as a primary cause of pre-eclampsia. However, it is not obvious how changes in implantation lead first to pre-eclampsia and then to long-term changes in risk of stroke and end-stage renal disease. In rat models of pre-eclampsia, ouabain treatment leads to symptoms of life-threatening hypertension [53]. Our theory is that hyper-spirolemia, secondary to inadequate fetal potassium, may be the proximate cause of the increased long-term incidence of congestive heart failure and/or end-stage renal failure.

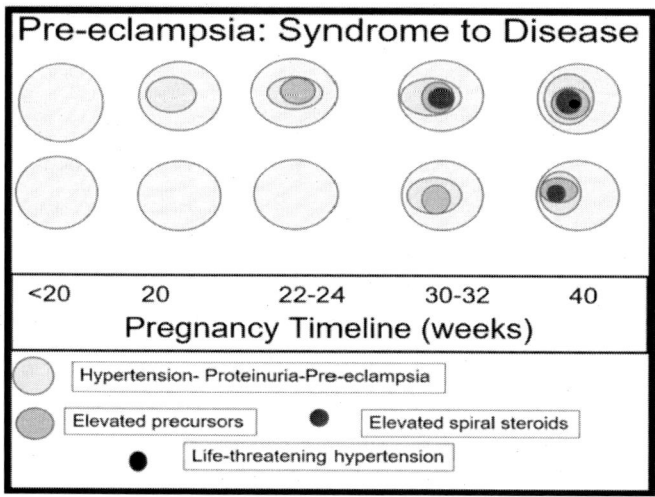

Figure 20. Pre-eclampsia and life-threatening hypertension.

Every year 50,000 women in the US experience life-threatening hypertension events during pregnancy and/or childbirth. Women are screened for gestational diabetes and thyroid disorders, but there is no, FDA approved, method for screening for gestational electrolyte disorders. We are proposing measurement of C313 and C329 as markers for gestational electrolyte disorders. There may be a benefit to combine the spiral steroid precursor assay with the current standard of care for other gestational diseases. Blood tests are already routinely drawn at 16 and 28 weeks of pregnancy and either time point might be a good opportunity to obtain blood samples to test potential markers for pre-eclampsia.

CONCLUSION

The first two sections of this chapter describe the discovery of spiral steroids. The discovery includes structure, function, synthesis, and application to diagnosis of human disease. There is no similar collection of data underlying the case for endogenous ouabain or marinobufagenin. Readers should make a careful review of the underlying data for any one of these compounds as mammalian cardiotonic steroids.

The second half of the chapter proposes elevated C313 and C329 as the proximate cause of pre-eclampsia in some patients. This feature divides patients into two groups: [a] a disease characterized by hypertension, proteinuria and elevated levels of spiral steroid precursors and [b] a stub syndrome characterized by normal levels of spiral steroid precursors, hypertension and proteinuria. The fact that the classical symptoms of pre-eclampsia are present in more than one disease may be the reason for the difficulty in development of therapeutic protocols.

Finally, elevated spiral steroids (hyper-spirolemia) may be a proximate cause of life-threatening hypertension during the 3rd trimester and may also be a factor in the increased long-term incidence of renal and heart disease in women who had pre-eclampsia.

ACKNOWLEDGMENTS

I specifically wish to recognize three very special colleagues: Dr. Ron Bochner, Dr. H. Leon Bradlow and Dr. Sandra Blethen (Chasalow).

Colleagues included, Dr. Kathryn King, LIJMC, Dr. Sharon Nachman, LIJMC, Dr. Gary Jarvis, VA Medical Center, San Francisco, CA and by Dr. Constance John, VA Medical Center, San Francisco, CA. Dr. John encouraged me and made laboratory space and equipment available. My two laboratory chiefs were Michael Davis and Lori Pierce-Cohen. Dr. Forbes Porter and Dr. Christopher Wassif of the NICHD provided serum samples from patients and obligate heterozygotes with Smith-Lemli-Opitz syndrome. Dr. Alisha Romano provided serum samples collected in the normal course of patient care.

Marvin Applets were used for drawing, displaying and characterizing chemical structures and reactions, Product Version 20.1 ChemAxon (https://www. Chemaxon.com).

Funding Statement

This research did not receive any specific grant from funding agencies in the public, commercial or not-for-profit sectors. Dr. Ron Bochner personally funded the pilot study of women with pre-eclampsia. The Smith-Lemli-Opitz Foundation funded the investigation of the patients with SLO syndrome. AMUR Research Corp funded most of the original investigations. Kerix funded the purification of the compounds with 23 carbon atoms and the investigation of the chemical formulas. This work was partially supported by the Research Service of the United States Department of Veterans Affairs. Current support is from IOMA LLC.

REFERENCES

[1] Szent-Gyorgyi A. (1985) Chemical physiology of contraction in body and heart muscle. Academic Press. New York, NY. (As cited in Labella FS. (1985) Endogenous digitalis-like factors: Introductory Remarks. *Fed Proc. 44*: 2780-2781.

[2] Walsh P, Crawford F, & Hawker CD. (1977) Measurement of digoxin by radioimmunoassay. *Annals of Clinical and Laboratory Science. 7*: 79-87.

[3] van Abbe R. (1982) Nurse cleared in infant deaths. *UPI Archives.* May 21.

[4] Hamlyn J, Blaustein M, Bova S, DuCharme D, Harris D, Mandel F, Mathews W, & Ludens J. (1991) Identification and characterization

of an ouabain-like compound from human plasma. *Proc Natl Acad Sci. 88*: 6259-6263.

[5] Blethen SL & Chasalow FI. (1989) Characterization of a digoxin-like material in salt-wasting congenital adrenal hyperplasia (CAH). *3rd Joint Meeting European Society for Pediatric Endocrinology/Lawson Wilkins Pediatric Endocrine Society.* Jerusalem, Israel.

[6] Giraud M, Naismith J687-696. (2000). The rhamnose pathway. *Current Opinion in Structural Biology.* 10: 687-696. doi.org/10.1016/S0959-440X(00)00145-7.

[7] Baecher S, Kroiss M, Fassnacht M, & Vogeser M. (2014) No endogenous ouabain is detectable in human plasma by ultrasensitive UPLC-MS/MS. *Clin Chim Acta,* 431: 87-9.

[8] Chasalow F & Pierce-Cohen L. (2018) Ionotropin is the mammalian digoxin-like material (DLM). It is a phosphocholine ester of a steroid with 23 carbon atoms. *Steroids 136:*63-75. doi: 10.1016/j.steroids.2018.03.001. Epub 2018 Mar.

[9] Smith DW, Lemli L, & Opitz M. (1964) A newly recognized syndrome of multiple congenital anomalies. *J Pediatrics.* 64: 210-217. Pubmed 14119520.

[10] Chasalow F, Blethen S, & Taysi K. (1985). Possible abnormalities of steroid secretion in children with Smith-Lemli-Opitz syndrome and their parents. *Steroids.* 46: 827-843.

[11] Bradlow H, Fleisher M, Breed C, & Chasalow F. (1990) Biochemical classification of patients with gross cystic breast disease. *N Y Acad Sci. 586*:12-16.

[12] Chasalow FI & Bradlow HL. (1990) Digoxin-like materials in human breast cyst fluids. *Ann N Y Acad Sci. 586*:107-16. doi: 10.1111/j.1749-6632.1990.tb17797.x. PubMed PMID: 2162647.

[13] Chasalow F. (2001). Phosphocholinate cardenolides. *US Patent 6,177,461 B1.*

[14] Chasalow F. (2000) Synthesis of DHEA-PC. Phospholipid drug derivatives. *US Patent 6,127,349.*

[15] Burstein S & Gut M. (1971) Biosynthesis of pregnenolone. *Recent Prog Horm Res.* 27:303-49. doi: 10.1016/b978-0-12-571127-2.50032-8. PMID: 4946132.

[16] Slominski A, Zmijewski M, Semak I, Sweatman T, Janjetovic Z, Li W, & Zjawiony J. (2008) Sequential metabolism of 7-dehydro-cholesterol to steroid 5,7-dienes in adrenal glands and its biological implication in the skin. *PLoS ONE* 4(2): e4309. doi: 10.1371/journal.pone.0004309.

[17] Slominski A, Ziawiony J, Wortsman J, Semak I, Stewart J, Pisarchik A, Steatman T, Marcos J, Dunbar C, & Tuckey R. (2004) A novel pathway for sequential transformation of 7-dehydro-cholesterol and expression of the P450 SCC system in mammalian skin. *Eur J Biochem.* 271: 4178-4188.

[18] Chasalow F. (2018) A new concept: Ionotropin May Be a Factor in Mobilization for [a] the Flight or Fight response and [b] Childbirth. *EC Paediatrics.* 7: 909-918. doi: 10.31080/ecpe.2018.07.00341

[19] Gibellini F & Smith T. (2010) The Kennedy Pathway – De Novo Synthesis of phosphatidyl ethanolamine and Phosphatidylcholine. IUBMB *Life* 62 (6): 414-428. doi: 10.1002/iub.337.

[20] Shackleton C, Roitman, E, Guo LW, Wilson WK, & Porter FD. (2002) Identification of 7(8) and 8(9) unsaturated adrenal steroid metabolites produced by patients with 7-dehydrosterol-delta-7-reductase deficiency (Smith-Lemli-Opitz Syndrome). *J Steroid Biochem Mol Biol.* 82: 225-32. Pubmed/12477489.

[21] Chasalow F & Blethen S. (2020) Steroid Metabolic Consequences of 7-Dehydrosterol Reductase Deficiency (SLO). *EC Paediatrics.* 9: 60-69. doi: 10.31080/ecpe.2020.09.00720.

[22] Chasalow F. (2019). Spiral Phosphocholine Steroids and DLM in Chicken Eggs (*Gallus domesticus*). *EC Paediatrics* 8: 01-12. doi: 10.31080/ecpe.2019.08.00593.

[23] Chasalow F. (2020). Phosphocholine Steroid Esters in Pacific Oysters (*Crassostrea gigas*). *EC Pediatrics* 9: 115-126. doi: 10.31080/ecpe.2020.09.00844.

[24] Bagrov A, Shapiro J, & Fedorova O. (2009). Endogenous Cardiotonic Steroids: Physiology, Pharmacology, and Novel Therapeutic Targets. *Pharmacological Reviews*. 61: 9-38.

[25] Füerstenwerth H. (2018). *Ouabain: A gift from paradise*. Amazon Publishing.

[26] Blaustein M. (2014) Why isn't endogenous ouabain more widely accepted? *Am J Physiol Heart Circ Physiology*. 307(5): H635-H639. doi: 10.1152/ajpeart.00402.2014.

[27] Nicholls MG, Lewis LK, Yandle TG, Lord G, McKinnon W, & Hilton PJ. (2009). Ouabain, a circulating hormone secreted by the adrenals, is pivotal in cardiovascular disease. Fact or fantasy? *J Hypertens*. 27(1): 3-8. doi: 10.1097/HJH.0b013e32831101d1.

[28] Tomaschitz A, Piecha G, Ritz E, Meinitzer A, Haas J, Pieske B, Wiecek A, Rus-Machan J, Toplak H, Marz W, Verheyen N, Gaksch M, Amrein K, Kraigher-KrainerE, Fahrleitner-Pammer A, & Pilz S. (2015) Marinobufagenin in essential hypertension and primary aldosteronism: A cardiotonic steroid with clinical and diagnostic implications. *Clin Exp Hypertens*, 37:108-15. doi: 10.3109/ 10641963.2014.913604.

[29] Chasalow F. (2018) A new concept for the regulation of electrolytes in pregnancy: the role of Ionotropin: The endogenous potassium sparing hormone. *Pediatrics (E-cronicon)*. 7(6): 527-532. doi:10. 31080/ecpe.2018.07.00267.

[30] Chasalow F. (2021) Spiral steroids during pregnancy. *The Endocrine Society*. Abstract # 6710. Poster Session P45.

[31] King K, Chasalow F, Faklis E, & Blethen S. (1994) Post-natal changes in growth hormone isoforms in preterm and term infants. *Endocrinol Metab I (Suppl B)*: 13.

[32] Nachman S, Chasalow F, Navaie-Waliser M, Blethen S, & Tropper P. (1996) Testing cord blood human chorionic gonadotropin as a surrogate marker for early identification of human immunodeficiency virus-1 infection in children. *J Perinatol* 16: 449-54. Pubmed 8979183.

[33] Chasalow F, & Blethen S. (1990) Characterization of digoxin-like material in human cord serum. *Ann N Y Acad Sci.* 591: 212-21. PMID: 2142872.

[34] Bizzarri C, Pedicelli S, Cappa M, & Cianfarani S. (2016) Water Balance and 'Salt Wasting' in the First Year of Life: The Role of Aldosterone-Signaling *Defects. Horm Res Paediatr.* 86: 143-153. doi:10.1159/000449057.

[35] Myatt L, & Roberts J. (2015) Preeclampsia: Syndrome or Disease. *Curr Hypertens Rep.* 17: 83. doi: 10.1007/s11906-015-0595-4.

[36] Ogge G, Chaiworapongsa T, Romero R, Hussein Y, Kusanovic J, Yeo L, Kim C, & Hassan S. (2011). Placental Lesions Associated with Maternal Underperfusion are more Frequent in Early-onset than in Late-onset Pre-eclampsia. *J Perinat Med 39*: 641-652. 25: doi:10.1515/JPM.2011.098.

[37] Ananthe CV, Keyes KM, & Warner RJ. (2013) Pre-eclampsia rates in United States 1980 to 2010: age-period-cohort analysis. *BMJ* 347: f6564. doi: https://doi.org/10.1136/bmj.f6564.

[38] Vikse B, Irgens L, Leivestad T, Skjaerven R, & Iversen B. (2008). Preeclampsia and the Risk of End-Stage Renal Disease. *N Engl J Med.* 359:800-9. doi: 10.1056/NEJMoa0706790.

[39] https://pre-eclampsia.org/long-term-impact-healthcare-providers. Dated July17,2020.

[40] Hahn S. (2015) Pre-eclampsia – will orphan drug status facilitate innovative biological therapies? *Frontiers in Surgery.* 2: article 7. doi:10.3389/fsurg.2015.00007.

[41] Estabrook G, Brown M, & Sargent I. (2011) The origins and end-organ consequence of pre-eclampsia. *Best Practice & Research Clinical Obstetrics and Gynaecology.* 25: 435-447.

[42] Poon L & Nicolaides K. (2014) Early Prediction of Pre-eclampsia. *Obstetrics and Gynecology International*: article ID 297397. doi:org/10.1155/2014/297397.

[43] Alberry M, Bills V, & Soothill P. (2011). Review: An update on pre-eclampsia prediction research. *The Obstetrician & Gynaecologist.* 13: 79-85.

[44] Graves S. (1987) The Possible role of Digitalislike Factors in Pregnancy-Induced Hypertension. *Hypertension 10 {suppl I}:* I-84-6.

[45] Chasalow F, John C, & Bochner R. (2019) Spiral steroids as potential markers for pre-eclampsia: a pilot study. *Steroids.* Nov. 151: 108466. doi:10.1016/j.steroids.2019.108466. Epub 2019 Jul 26. PubMed PMID: 31351941.

[46] Wu P, van den Berg C, Alfirevic Z, O'Brien S, Rothlisberger M, Baker P, Kenny L, Kublickiene K, & Duvekot J. (2015) Early Pregnancy Biomarkers in Pre-Eclampsia: A Systematic Review and Meta-Analysis. *International Journal of Molecular Sciences.* 16: 23035-23056. doi:10.3390/ijms160923035.

[47] Reynolds T. (2010) The triple test as a screening technique for Down syndrome: reliability and relevance. *International Journal of Women's Health.* 2: 83-88. PMC2971727.

[48] Grill S, Rusterholz C, Zanetti-Dallenbach R, Tercanli S, Holzgreve W, Hahn S, & Lapaire O. (2009) Potential markers of preeclampsia – a review. *Reproductive Biology and Endocrinology.* 7:70. doi:10.1186/1477-7827-7-70.

[49] Leslie K, Thilaganathan B, & Papageorghiou A. (2011) *Best Practice & Research Clinical Obstetrics and Gynaecology.* Early prediction and prevention of pre-eclampsia. 25: 343-354. doi:10.1016/j.bpobgyn.2011.01.002.

[50] Costa F. Murth P, Keogh R, & Woodrow N. (2011) Early Screening for preeclampsia. *The Revista Brasileira de Ginecologia e Obstetr′ıcia,* 33, 367–375. [*The Brazilian Journal of Gynecology and Obstetrics*]

[51] Lupoglazoff J, Jacoz-Aigrain E, Guyot B, Chappey O, & Blot P. (1993) Endogenous digoxin-like immunoreactivity during pregnancy and at birth. *Br J clin Pharmac.* 35: 251-254.

[52] Fedorva O, Tapilskaya N, Bzhelyansky A, Frolova E, Nikitina R, Reznik V, Kashkin V, & Bagrov A. (2010) Interaction of Digibind with endogenous cardiotonic steroids from pre-eclamptic placentae. *J. Hypertens* 28: 361-366. doi: 10.1097/HJH.0b013e328333226c.

[53] Yuan C. Manunta P, Hamlyn J, Chen S, Bohen E, Yeun J, Haddy F, Pamnani M. (1993). Long-term Ouabain Administration Produces Hypertension in Rats. *Hypertension*. 22:178-187.

In: Eclampsia
Editor: Sharon Wright
ISBN: 978-1-53619-574-3
© 2021 Nova Science Publishers, Inc.

Chapter 3

POSTPARTUM PRE-ECLAMPSIA

Igor Lakhno[1],, MD, PhD, DSc and Kemine Uzel[2]*

[1]Obstetrics and gynecology department,
Kharkiv Medical Academy of Postgraduate Education,
Kharkiv, Ukraine
[2]Erzincan Binali Yildirim University
Mengucek Gazi Training and Research Hospital,
Department of Gynecology and Obstetrics,
Erzincan, Turkey

ABSTRACT

Pre-eclampsia occurs only in humans during the second half of pregnancy or the postpartum period. It is known to be featured by the development of arterial hypertension and multiple organ failure. The main role of the placental lesions in the pathogenetic scenario was shown. The high level of perinatal pathology is a reason for the continual search in the field. Almost a third of eclampsia occurs in the postpartum period. The pre-eclamptic patients require thorough monitoring of blood pressure and administration of antihypertensive drugs in the puerperium.

---

* Corresponding Author's E-mail: igorlakhno71@gmail.com.

The pathogenesis and the management of the developed de novo postpartum pre-eclampsia have not been sufficiently studied. The greatest risk of brain stroke after delivery remains for 10 days. It is very important to start the antihypertensives in time. „First-line" drugs should be used not later than 30 - 60 minutes from the time of severe pre-eclampsia diagnosing to prevent intracranial hemorrhage. Labetalol or hydralazine should be used to reduce blood pressure. Sublingual administration of nifedipine may also be considered as „first-line" therapy. The use of magnesium sulfate is necessary for the prevention of seizures in patients with severe pre-eclampsia. In the case of eclampsia, a solution of magnesium sulfate is being administered intravenously at a loading dose of 4 - 5g for 15 - 20 minutes and then the infusion is being continued at a dose of 1 g per hour throughout the day. Uterine curettage is also a possible intervention for reducing blood pressure in women with pre-eclampsia.

The clinical case of a systemic inflammatory response syndrome that occurred in a postpartum woman with mild pre-eclampsia is given. Postpartum endometritis, which was caused by group B streptococcus, should have played a triggering role in the progression of preeclampsia. The problem of poly chemical resistance has led to the inability of traditional antimicrobial agents to prevent the dissemination of infection after curettage. The systemic inflammatory response syndrome has contributed to the increased severity of preeclampsia and the development of multiple organ failure.

Pre-eclampsia (PE) is a disease found only in humans during II half of gestation or after delivery that is featured by arterial hypertension and may develop multiple organ failure. PE is one of the main reasons for maternal morbidity and mortality. Atherosclerosis, hypertension, coronary heart disease, and brain stroke are the consequences of PE in the further lifetime [18]. This gestational pathology is associated with arterial hypertension, proteinuria, and end-organ malfunction. The placental ischemic syndrome was proved to be the initial stage of the systemic vasculopathy in PE. Increased levels of the placental pro-inflammatory cytokines, vasoconstrictors, and lipid peroxidation products are known to be involved in the pathogenetic scenario of PE. Endothelial dysfunction is the central event in the end-organ failure [29]. The systemic inflammatory response syndrome (SIRS) reflects the severity of PE but it has no clinical equivalents in mild and moderate pre-eclamptic patients [4]. SIRS is a satellite for severe PE or eclampsia and different types of shock. Thus, non-infectious inflammation is a major component of PE. A possible reason for this inflammatory response in the second half of gestation could be associated with the HLA-incompatibility between the mother and the fetus, the fetal DNA, the products of ischemic necrosis, or apoptosis of the syncytiotrophoblast, etc. [14].

The lack of evidence makes the possible role of infection in the origin and progression of PE rather unpopular [15, 20]. A higher incidence of PE occurs in pregnant women with urinary tract infection, periodontal disease, bacterial vaginosis, and other comorbidities. Any maternal infection was associated with a two-fold higher risk of PE in one systematic review [11]. The relevant issue is whether infectious agents are involved in the pathogenesis of multiple organ failure in PE?

Almost one-third of all cases of PE are known to occur postpartum (within 48 hours after delivery). Half of the intracranial hemorrhages could happen in the puerperium [1, 5, 28]. Thus, the pre-eclamptic women should receive antihypertensives and require monitoring. Since PE is known to increase the risk of cardiovascular disease, consultations with cardiologists or neurologists are often required for pre-eclamptic women [2, 30]. But the majority of patients hope for complete recovery just after the delivery. That is why the delay in antihypertensive drug prescription counteracts the restoration and rehabilitation [8]. Nowadays, there are a lot of issues in the management of pre-eclamptic patients.

The lack of trophoblastic invasion is known to be a triggering event in the pathogenetic scenario of PE. The imbalance between angiogenic and antiangiogenic substances disturbs the invasion. Chorionic or placental ischemia induces the synthesis and releases into systemic circulation proinflammatory cytokines, the products of peroxidation, and vasoconstrictors [14]. The generalized vascular spasm is associated with endothelial malfunction. Oxidative stress causes the development of dyslipidemia that stimulates peroxidation [13]. The lipid vesicles in placental vessels depositing – so-called atherosis enhances the placental ischemia. The thrombotic events in the placental site could be an additional pathogenetic pathway for ischemia. Therefore, PE has two stages by C. W. Redman: preclinical one associated with failed placentation, and the maternal syndrome [1]. C. W. Redman is an eminent person in the field. He had investigated the role of SIRS in the pathogenesis of PE and separated early-onset (before 32 weeks), and late-onset PE. Late-onset PE is mainly a maternal disease without evident fetal growth restriction. The proteinuria was ruled out from severe PE criteria according to the decision of ACOG [3]. The Finnish Pre-eclampsia Consortium showed that this recommendation contributed to the improvement of the sensitivity and specificity of PE diagnosing [16]. But are there any evident differences between PE before delivery and developed de novo postpartum?

The pathogenesis of the postpartum PE is not known completely. The immune malfunction could be involved in the scenario [6]. The alarmin imbalance was found to participate in the development of PE. Alarmins are endogenous molecular complexes synthesized in non-apoptotic tissue lesions. The increased level of uric acid was detected in women with early- or late-onset PE. The elevated concentration of amphoterin was found in women with postpartum PE. This alarmin substance is known to be elevated in sepsis (SIRS) [12]. The differences in a cellular branch of immunity in patients with early-onset, late-onset, and postpartum PE were found. The growth of the capacity of lymphatic and monocytic cells was detected in the conventional pre-delivery development of PE. The increased quantity of granulocytes – NK-cells and the elevated placental CD45+ cells with the predominance of CD163+ cells in postpartum PE were found. The lymphatic and monocytic infiltration was a repercussion of the pre-delivery onset of PE [4]. The pro-inflammatory changes were mutual for all types of PE without any relation to the time of origin. The immune malfunction is known to be involved in the placental lesions. The investigation of the inflammatory immune pathways of PE could contribute to the development of novel methods for postpartum PE prevention.

The placental morphometry findings showed that the placental weight was similar in late-onset and postpartum PE. But the degree of the decidual inflammatory changes was higher in postpartum PE. The maximal quantity of placental infarctions and the signs of preterm placental maturation was found in early-onset PE [12]. These findings support the placental theory of PE development. Maternal diseases and external negative stimuli may develop postpartum PE. The peculiarities of labor could contribute to the development or progression of PE.

The analysis for postpartum PE risk factors in women with normotension during pregnancy was performed. It was found that late maternal age (> 40 years), Latin nationality, obesity, and gestational diabetes mellitus are linked with postpartum PE [5]. The possible role of fluid load, oxytocin infusion, and neuraxial analgesia in the development of postpartum PE was investigated. The logistic regression showed the prognostic value of body mass index (BMI) > 30kg/m2 at early pregnancy, and crystalloids infusion during labor [10, 21, 25]. Therefore, postpartum PE has a similar to metabolic syndrome pathogenesis or could be the result of fluid overload during delivery.

PE is featured by hypovolemia and increased vascular permeability. Fluid overload may cause kidney damage as a result of renin-angiotensin-aldosterone system suppression and an elevated level of antiangiogenic substances [9, 27]. The initial hypovolemia and the increased vascular permeability may contribute to the dissemination of the crystalloids into the extravascular space. But the pathogenesis of postpartum PE developed within 48 hours after delivery or 6 weeks later is quite different. The recent findings supported the possible role of pregestational BMI > 25kg/m2, cesarean section, assisted reproductive technologies, chronic inflammatory kidney disease, hypothyreosis, and elevated blood pressure at the first antenatal visit before 14 weeks of gestation in the development of postpartum PE. Thus, the most realistic approach to the prevention of postpartum PE is bodyweight reduction during preconception. The use of low dose acetylsalicylic acid is evident only for early-onset PE [1].

The usage of antihypertensive drugs and blood pressure monitoring should be continued after delivery in pre-eclamptic patients. The brain hypoperfusion persists to stay in PE. The autoregulation of the intracranial hemodynamics is suppressed [17]. The blood pressure should be under strict control within 2 weeks postpartum according to NICE recommendations [8]. The most accurate blood pressure measurement is necessary 3 - 5 days after delivery. The rise of blood pressure is possible at this time. The antihypertensives should be prescribed in case of blood pressure elevation up to 150/100 or even higher. The treatment should be completed if blood pressure is lower than 130/80 [1, 23]. The regimen of drug dose reduction is still an issue. ACOG recommends blood pressure monitoring within 72 hours postpartum in maternal clinic and continuation of this control during 7-10 days of puerperium [1]. The data was supported by the American National database on the healthcare cost for repeated hospitalization [30]. The dataset included more than 1 million deliveries. More than one thousand and five hundred cases of intracranial hemorrhages were found amongst the total study population. Only 14.2% of women had PE and 4.4% –chronic arterial hypertension. No data on any prodromes of the hypertension was found in 81.4%. The majority of brain stroke cases occurred within 10 days postpartum. The diagnosed PE or chronic arterial hypertension were found to increase the risk of brain stroke postpartum by 74%.

The timely onset of the usage of antihypertensives is of great significance in the case of postpartum PE manifestation. The "first line" drugs should be prescribed not later than 30 - 60 minutes after the initial blood pressure elevation. This intervention is necessary for the prevention of intracranial hemorrhage. Labetalol or hydralazine are routinely used for the quick restoration of blood pressure. Labetalol is the only β-blocker with evident internal sympathomimetic activity. Thus, this drug does not decrease cardiac output. It is of great value in hypovolemia. Bronchial asthma is a principal contraindication for labetalol [26]. The use of calcium channel antagonists is less investigated. But sublingual nifedipine could be also thought of as "first-line" therapy. There is no sufficient information on the benefits of labetalol compared to nifedipine usage [23]. Any severe pre-eclamptic patient with a lack of labetalol, hydralazine, or nifedipine efficiency should be admitted to the resuscitation unit for mutual management with the anesthesiologist. The management of severe PE requires the use of a multidisciplinary approach and ophthalmologists, cardiologists, neurologists, and nephrologists are invited for teamwork.

The magnesium sulfate solution should be used for the prevention of convulsions in severe PE. The intravenous administration of 4 - 5g of magnesium sulfate should be performed within 15 - 20 minutes. The infusion of 1g per hour of magnesium sulfate will be continued for 24 hours [31]. Besides the anticonvulsant effect, magnesium sulfate has anti-inflammatory and vasorelaxation action. Since the usage of magnesium sulfate contributes to the accumulation of magnesium ions, the level of blood serum magnesium is necessary. This monitoring is included in the Glasgow scale calculation (not more than 15). The rate of respiration (more than 12 per minute), the check for tendon reflexes grading, and monitoring of diuresis (more than 30ml/hour) should be performed. The infusion must be stoped in case of any sign of magnesium overdose. The injection of calcium gluconate and the analysis for blood serum magnesium should be performed [2].

Calcium channel blockers, β-blockers, vasodilators, and other drugs are used for the prolonged control of blood pressure. There's no difference between clonidine vs captopril in their efficiency [5]. The benefits of using indapamide vs methyldopa were not found [8]. The usage of loop diuretics is limited because of insufficient information on their safety [9]. Furthermore, thiazide diuretics are not used in the UK during breastfeeding. Methyldopa or reserpine should not be prescribed during the lactation period [21]. Breastfeeding is known to decrease the risk of cardiovascular disease in pre-eclamptic women [7]. The prescription of furosemide was found to reduce the necessity for the additional usage of antihypertensives [26]. The application of L-arginine did not provide any benefits to the users of antihypertensive drugs [8]. The further investigation of carperitide efficiency in pre-eclamptic postpartum patients is of great prospect [31].

The uterine curettage is also known as a possible intervention for the reduction of blood pressure in PE. The use of curettage is similar to sublingual nifedipine application according to their antihypertensive therapeutic potentials. Since placental and decidual tissue is known to play a triggering role in PE, its evacuation during curettage is rather rational. But curettage may increase the risk of uterine perforation, the dissemination of infection in case of endometritis, and narcosis complications [22]. Therefore, curettage should be performed during cesarean section [8].

The above data demonstrate the lack of possibility to prevent all possible complications of postpartum PE. Since postpartum PE is atypical, the management should be individualized. The clinical case of postpartum PE and SIRS captures this thesis [19].

A pregnant woman aged 30 years was admitted to the division of maternal-fetal medicine at 24 weeks of gestation. She had irregular antenatal visits, which revealed no abnormality. She had blood pressure (BP) of 140/90, a pulse of 82 per minute, and a normal body temperature at the admission office. She had no prodromes suggestive of arterial hypertension. Laboratory findings were unremarkable (hemoglobin, leukocytes, platelet count, serum aspartate aminotransaminase, serum alanine aminotransaminase, serum urea, serum creatinine concentration, and coagulation profile were normal) with a trace of proteinuria in urinalysis. Bacterial vaginosis was diagnosed. She had a mild PE, an early fetal growth restriction, and a post-cesarean uterine scar. No maternal internal diseases were known. The maternal condition was stable but fetal demise occurred. Ceftriaxone injections were started, as is our standard practice for intrauterine death. Labor was induced by an intracervical insertion of laminaria. A dead female fetus of 510g was born. Curettage was performed because of the uterine scar and the partly retained placenta. The patient additionally received 2g of ceftriaxone and 500mg of metronidazole intravenously. BP was 130/95, urinary protein in a single portion – 0.015g/l, hematological indices were normal. The postpartum woman complained of headaches, visual disturbances, and mild muscle spasms within 8 hours. BP consequently jumped to 210/130, proteinuria to 6.5g/l. These data and the absence of any internal disease in the history supported severe PE. She did not have any generalized seizures. The patient received 4 g of MgSO4 within 20 minutes intravenously as a loading dose and then an infusion of MgSO4 was maintained at a rate of 1g/hour for 24 hours. An infusion of 60mg of hydralazine was also done at a rate of 2 - 10mg/hour depending on the BP and pulse rate. BP fell to

150/90. The data of the bio-impedance cardiography supported the hypokinetic type of the central hemodynamics with end-organ hypoperfusion. The patient received antihypertensives, antimicrobial agents, and infusion therapy. An enlarged hepatic volume was found at the end of the first day of the postpartum period, but the level of serum aspartate aminotransaminase and serum alanine aminotransaminase was not increased considerably and the platelet count was stable. Therefore, HELLP syndrome was excluded. Later on, within 1 day acute renal failure developed (serum creatinine concentration was 2.2mg/dl). A positive test for procalcitonin, an increased level of the C-reactive protein and leukocytosis were detected at the same time. Therefore, the patient had puerperal sepsis. The uterus was enlarged and painful, the discharge was bloody and purulent. The microbiological investigation of the cervical culture revealed significant growth of group B Streptococcus with the only determining sensitivity to vancomycin. Any agents of sexually transmitted diseases were not detected by a polymerase chain reaction. Blood and urine cultures were negative. Rebound tenderness was found in the lower abdomen. Since endometritis and pelvic peritonitis were diagnosed the patient was operated on. A hysterectomy was performed on the third day after delivery. After several days, the condition of the postpartum patient improved. The level of BP was reduced within 10 days. She was sent home in 14 days. A histological investigation supported the purulent endometritis.

Bacterial vaginosis is associated with a higher incidence of chronic endometritis [11]. The abnormal uteroplacental hemodynamics caused by group B streptococcus-associated endometritis possibly played a triggering role in the development of PE in this case. Since shallow trophoblastic invasion into the spiral arteries is known as a reason for the placental ischemic syndrome, the worsening PE development could be associated with the microbial inhabitants of the genital tract [24]. The problem of resistance to antimicrobial agents contributed to the dramatic outcome. PE typically reduces but not progresses after pregnancy is terminated [1, 3], – our case is unusual in that PE progressed postpartum, possibly related to the inflammatory environment. The decreased intraabdominal pressure after delivery is known to be one of the most significant factors contributing to the reestablishment of hemodynamics [3, 31]. The application of ceftriaxone and metronidazole was ineffective and could not counteract the dissemination of infection after curettage. The clinical manifestation of prodromal events of eclampsia reflected the SIRS. Therefore, the infection likely enhanced the severity of PE and contributed to the development of multiple organ failure. Since the uterus is the source of sepsis, the hysterectomy enables avoiding general peritonitis and septic shock. The consequent recovery was rather logical.

Therefore, infectious inflammation could be involved in PE pathogenesis and contribute to the progressive severity of the disease even in the puerperium. PE is still an enigma. An obstetrician should become more vigilant to prevent complications.

REFERENCES

[1] ACOG Committee Opinion No. 767 Summary: Emergent Therapy for Acute-Onset, Severe Hypertension during Pregnancy and the Postpartum Period. *Obstet. Gynecol.*, 2019; 133(2):409 - 412.

[2] Al-Safi, Z., Imudia, A. N., Filetti, L. C., Hobson, D. T., Bahado-Singh, R. O., Awonuga, A. O. Delayed postpartum preeclampsia and eclampsia: Demographics, clinical course, and complications. *Obstet. Gynecol.*, 2011; 118(5):1102 - 7.

[3] American College of Obstetricians and Gynecologists, Task Force on Hypertension in Pregnancy. Hypertension in pregnancy. Report of the American College of Obstetricians and Gynecologists' Task Force on Hypertension in Pregnancy. *Obstet. Gynecol.*, 2013; 122(5): 1122 - 31.

[4] Ann-Charlotte, I. Inflammatory mechanisms in preeclampsia. *Pregnancy Hypertens.*, 2013; 3(2):58.

[5] Bigelow, C. A., Pereira, G. A., Warmsley, A., Cohen, J., Getrajdman, C., Moshier, E., Paris, J., Bianco, A., Factor, S. H., Stone, J. Risk factors for new-onset late postpartum preeclampsia in women

without a history of preeclampsia. *Am. J. Obstet. Gynecol.,* 2014; 210(4):338 e1 - 8.

[6] Brien, M. E., Boufaied, I., Soglio, D. D., Rey, E., Leduc, L., Girard, S. Distinct inflammatory profile in preeclampsia and postpartum preeclampsia reveal unique mechanisms. *Biol. Reprod.,* 2019; 100(1):187 - 194.

[7] Burgess, A., McDowell, W., Ebersold, S. Association between Lactation and Postpartum Blood Pressure in Women with Preeclampsia. *MCN Am. J. Matern. Child Nurs.,* 2019; 44(2):86 - 93.

[8] Cairns, A. E., Pealing, L., Duffy, J. M. N. et al. Postpartum management of hypertensive disorders of pregnancy: Late postpartum eclampsia. *J. Obstet. Gynaecol.,* 2012; 32(3):264 - 6. a systematic review. BMJ Open, 2017;7:e018696.

[9] Clark, T. P. Late-onset postpartum preeclampsia: A case study. *The Nurse practitioner,* 2014; 39(7): 34 - 42.

[10] Cohen, J., Vaiman, D., Sibai, B. M., Haddad, B. Blood pressure changes during the first stage of labor and for the prediction of early postpartum preeclampsia: A prospective study. *European Journal of Obstetrics, Gynecology, and Reproductive Biology,* 2015; 184: 103 - 7.

[11] Conde-Aqudelo, A., Villar, J., Lindheimer, M. Maternal infection and risk of preeclampsia: Systematic review and metaanalysis. *Am. J. Obstet. Gynecol.,* 2008; 198(1): – P. 7 - 22.

[12] Ditisheim, A., Sibai, B., Tatevian, N. Placental Findings in Postpartum Preeclampsia: A Comparative Retrospective Study. *Am. J. Perinatol.,* 2019 doi: 10.1055/s-0039-1692716.

[13] Elliot, M. G. Oxidative stress and the evolutionary origins of preeclampsia. *J. Reprod. Immunol.,* 2016; 114:75 - 80.

[14] Friedman, A. M., Cleary, K. L. Prediction and prevention of ischemic placental disease. *Semin. Perinatol.,* 2014; 38 (3): 177 - 182.

[15] Herrera, J. A., Chaudhuri, G., Lopez-Jaramillo, P. Is infection a major risk factor for preeclampsia? *Med. Hypotheses,* 2001; 57 (3): 393 - 7.

[16] Jääskeläinen, T., Heinonen, S., Hämäläinen, E., Pulkki, K., Romppanen, J., Laivuori, H. FINNPEC. Impact of obesity on angiogenic and inflammatory markers in the Finnish Genetics of Pre-eclampsia Consortium (FINNPEC) cohort. *Int. J. Obes., (Lond).* 2019; 43(5):1070 - 1081.
[17] Janzarik, W. G., Jacob, J., Katagis, E., Markfeld-Erol, F., Sommerlade, L., Wuttke, M., Reinhard, M. Preeclampsia postpartum: Impairment of cerebral autoregulation and reversible cerebral hyperperfusion. *Pregnancy Hypertens.,* 2019; 17:121 - 126.
[18] Kalafat, E., Thilaganathan, B. Cardiovascular origins of preeclampsia. *Curr. Opin. Obstet. Gynecol.,* 2017; 29(6):383 - 389.
[19] Lakhno, I. V. Systemic Inflammatory Response Syndrome as a Reason for the Multiple Organ Failure in a Postpartum Pre-eclamptic Patient. *J. South Asian Feder. Obst. Gynae.,* 2018; 10(3):215 - 217.
[20] Lopez-Jaramillo, P., Herrera, J. A., Arenas-Mantilla, M., Jáuregui, I. E., Mendoza, M. A. Subclinical infection as a cause of inflammation in preeclampsia. *Am. J. Ther.,* 2008; 15 (4): 373 - 6.
[21] Matthys, L. A., Coppage, K. H., Lambers, D. S., Barton, J. R., Sibai, B. M. Delayed postpartum preeclampsia: an experience of 151 cases. *Am. J. Obstet. Gynecol.,* 2004; 190(5):1464 - 6.
[22] Mc Lean, G., Reyes, O., Velarde, R. Effects of postpartum uterine curettage in the recovery from Preeclampsia/Eclampsia. A randomized, controlled trial. *Pregnancy Hypertens.,* 2017; 10: 64 - 69.
[23] Odigboegwu, O., Pan, L. J., Chatterjee, P. Use of Antihypertensive Drugs during Preeclampsia. *Front. Cardiovasc. Med.,* 2018; 5:50.
[24] Rustveld, L. O., Kelsey, S. F., Sharma, R. Association between maternal infections and preeclampsia: A systematic review of epidemiologic studies. *Matern. Child Health J.,* 2008 Mar.; 12(2): – P. 223 - 42.
[25] Skurnik, G., Hurwitz, S., McElrath, T. F., Tsen, L. C., Duey, S., Saxena, A. R., Karumanchi, A., Rich-Edwards, J. W., Seely, E. W. Labor therapeutics and BMI as risk factors for postpartum

preeclampsia: A case-control study. *Pregnancy Hypertens.*, 2017; 10:177 - 181.

[26] Smith, G. N., Pudwell, J., Saade, G. R. Impact of the New American Hypertension Guidelines on the Prevalence of Postpartum Hypertension. *Am. J. Perinatol.*, 2019; 36(4):440 - 442.

[27] Takaoka, S., Ishii, K., Taguchi, T., Kakubari, R., Muto, H., Mabuchi, A., Yamamoto, R., Hayashi, S., Mitsuda, N. Clinical features and antenatal risk factors for postpartum-onset hypertensive disorders. *Hypertens. Pregnancy,* 2016:1 - 10.

[28] Too, G., Wen, T., Boehme, A. K., Miller, E. C., Leffert, L. R., Attenello, F. J., Mack, W. J., D'Alton, M. E., Friedman, A. M. Timing and Risk Factors of Postpartum Stroke. *Obstet. Gynecol.*, 2018; 131(1):70 - 78.

[29] Wang, P. H., Yang, M. J., Chen, C. Y., Chao, H. T. Endothelial cell dysfunction and preeclampsia. *J. Chin. Med. Assoc.*, 2015; 78(6): 321 - 2.

[30] Verhaegen, J., Peeters, F., Debois, P., Jacquemyn, Y. Posterior reversible encephalopathy syndrome as a complication of pre-eclampsia in the early postpartum period. *BMJ Case Rep.*, 2019; 12(7). pii: e228954.

[31] Yancey, L. M., Withers, E., Bakes, K., Abbott, J. Postpartum preeclampsia: emergency department presentation and management. *The Journal of Emergency Medicine*, 2011; 40(4):380 - 4.

INDEX

#

21-hydroxylase, 66, 92
7-dehydro-cholesterol, 78, 87, 109

A

acute renal failure, 123
adrenal gland, 109
age, viii, 2, 5, 8, 9, 18, 19, 22, 23, 31, 33, 38, 58, 65, 68, 111, 119
aldosterone, 85, 87, 90, 94, 102, 103, 104, 119
amniotic fluid, 90, 102, 104
androgens, 67, 83
anesthesiologist, 120
antibody, 68
anticoagulant, 50
anticoagulation, 47
anticonvulsant, 121
antihypertensive drugs, ix, 115, 119, 121
antiphospholipid syndrome, 40
aphasia, 5, 17, 26, 28, 33, 42, 44, 45
arterial hypertension, ix, 115, 116, 120, 122
arterioles, 33, 34, 56
atoms, 67, 68, 74, 78, 79, 82, 83, 84, 99

B

B12, 81
basal ganglia, 42, 43
bilateral, 10, 14, 15, 46
bile acids, 75
biochemistry, viii, 63, 90, 94
biomarkers, 95
biopsy, 93
biosynthesis, ix, 64
bleeding, 39
blindness, vii, viii, 2, 3, 4, 5, 6, 7, 8, 10, 11, 17, 26, 27, 28, 31, 32, 33, 36, 37, 44, 51, 53, 55, 59
blood, ix, 4, 6, 30, 31, 32, 33, 34, 35, 36, 37, 39, 40, 43, 47, 49, 87, 89, 90, 95, 103, 105, 110, 115, 116, 119, 120, 121, 122
blood flow, 34, 43, 89
blood pressure, ix, 6, 30, 31, 32, 33, 34, 35, 36, 43, 47, 49, 90, 95, 103, 115, 116, 119, 120, 121, 122
blood vessels, 35

blood-brain barrier, 4, 32, 43
brain, ix, 14, 31, 34, 35, 36, 37, 38, 39, 41, 42, 43, 45, 46, 49, 60, 116, 119
brain damage, 38
brain stem, 39, 43
breast cancer, 88
breastfeeding, 121

C

caesarean section, 7, 12, 18, 22, 26, 41
capillary, 35, 41, 43, 102
carbon atoms, viii, 63, 67, 72, 74, 75, 76, 77, 78, 79, 81, 82, 83, 84, 92, 99, 107, 108
cardiac output, 120
cardiotonic, 64, 66, 68, 82, 83, 85, 90, 95, 103, 106, 110, 113
cardiovascular disease, 56, 110, 117, 121
cation, 68, 73, 90, 93, 98, 99
CDP-serine, 80, 81
cell death, 38
central nervous system, 37
cerebellum, 39, 43
cerebral arteries, 32, 34, 39
cerebral blood flow, 32, 34, 35, 36, 59
cerebral cortex, 34
cerebral function, 5
cesarean section, 119, 122
chemical, ix, 67, 68, 73, 74, 107, 116
chemical structures, 107
children, 93, 99, 108, 110
cholesterol, 78, 87, 109
circulation, 4, 34, 35, 43, 55, 93, 95, 99, 117
clinical presentation, 42
clinical symptoms, 104
clinical syndrome, 3
coagulation profile, 6, 122
coagulopathy, 39, 40
co-enzyme A, 78, 81

complications, vii, viii, 1, 2, 3, 4, 5, 7, 8, 9, 10, 11, 12, 17, 18, 19, 22, 23, 26, 28, 30, 31, 32, 34, 40, 43, 45, 49, 51, 54, 122, 124
composition, 68, 74, 75, 84, 92
compounds, 67, 68, 70, 71, 77, 78, 81, 82, 83, 86, 106, 107
condensation, 78, 80, 81, 99
congenital adrenal hyperplasia, 108
congestive heart failure, 82, 105
consciousness, 5, 11, 18, 34, 42
control group, 22, 100, 102
coronary heart disease, 116
CT scan, 13, 14, 16, 28, 38, 39, 43, 45, 46
Cxxx, 67, 80, 81
cyst, 69, 85, 88, 108
cytokines, 116, 117

D

deaths, 3, 30, 48, 52, 53, 60, 107
deficiency, 35, 40, 66, 81, 87, 88, 109
deficit, 5, 7, 12, 24, 48
detachment, 5, 11, 27, 44
detectable, 68, 78, 103, 108
developing countries, 41, 48
DHEA-phosphocholine ester, 71, 72
diastolic blood pressure, viii, 2, 18, 23, 24, 32, 33, 49
diastolic pressure, 6, 32
diffusion, 84, 85, 86, 88, 96
digi-bind, 103
digoxin toxicity, 103
digoxin-like materials (DLM), 64, 65, 66, 69, 78, 83, 85, 87, 88, 93, 95, 96, 108, 109
disease progression, 103
diseases, ix, 31, 60, 63, 68, 102, 105, 119, 122
disorder, 30, 43, 104
drugs, ix, 47, 85, 86, 116, 120, 121

E

E313, 80, 81
eclampsia, v, vii, viii, ix, 1, 2, 3, 4, 5, 6, 7, 8, 9, 10, 12, 18, 19, 21, 22, 23, 24, 25, 26, 30, 31, 32, 33, 34, 35, 36, 37, 38, 39, 40, 43, 44, 48, 49, 51, 52, 53, 54, 55, 56, 58, 59, 60, 63, 65, 94, 95, 99, 103, 104, 105, 106, 115, 116, 117, 124, 125, 126
eggs, 82, 109
electrolyte, 68, 84, 86, 88, 89, 94, 96, 105
emergency, 3, 12, 51, 127
encephalopathy, 4, 31, 36, 54, 55, 56, 58, 127
endothelial dysfunction, 44
end-stage renal disease, 105
epithelial sodium channels (ENaC), 85
ester, 64, 67, 71, 72, 78, 85, 108
evidence, ix, 12, 44, 49, 50, 64, 71, 78, 85, 89, 104, 117
extravasation, 35, 36, 43
Exxx, 67, 80, 81

F

facial palsy, viii, 2, 5, 10, 17, 28, 29, 33, 44
fetal calf serum, 90, 92, 102
fetal demise, 122
fetal growth, 118, 122
fluid, 35, 41, 43, 68, 69, 89, 102, 119
Food and Drug Administration (FDA), 65, 94, 105
function, viii, 5, 6, 55, 56, 63, 64, 65, 67, 81, 83, 84, 85, 86, 87, 92, 93, 95, 102, 103, 106

G

gestation, 3, 5, 12, 45, 64, 99, 101, 116, 119, 122
gestational age, 65, 90, 94, 96, 104
gestational diabetes, 105, 119
Global Alliance for the Prevention of Prematurity and Stillbirth (GAPPS), 65, 96
glycoside, 66, 67, 82, 90, 103
growth, 93, 94, 110, 118, 123
growth hormone, 93, 110

H

hCG, 93
headache, 4, 22, 26, 36, 42, 45, 50
health, 49, 51, 53
health care, 51
health care professionals, 51
heart disease, 10, 94, 106
hemiparesis, viii, 2, 5, 10, 17, 26, 28, 29, 33, 42, 45
hemiplegia, viii, 2, 5, 10, 11, 17, 26, 28, 29, 32, 33, 45
hemorrhage, ix, 57, 58, 116, 120
hemorrhagic stroke, 4
hepatic failure, 3, 31
high blood pressure, 35, 94
history, 3, 6, 8, 37, 95, 122, 125
Hmax, 74
hormones, viii, 63, 64, 65, 67, 85, 86, 88, 91, 92, 94, 96, 102
Hreq, 74
human, 66, 68, 69, 71, 82, 85, 102, 106, 108, 110, 111
human chorionic gonadotropin, 110
human immunodeficiency virus, 110
hyper-spirolemia, 65, 88, 90, 105, 106
hypertension, viii, 3, 6, 30, 32, 33, 35, 36, 38, 39, 40, 43, 46, 47, 48, 49, 55, 56, 60, 63, 64, 65, 88, 89, 90, 94, 101, 104, 105, 106, 110, 116, 120
hypovolemia, 119, 120
hysterectomy, 123, 124

I

immunoreactivity, 112
implantation, 95, 102, 105
incidence, 8, 31, 37, 41, 48, 102, 105, 106, 117, 123
infants, 65, 66, 68, 87, 93, 94, 110
infarction, 36, 37, 39, 41, 42, 45
infection, ix, 41, 93, 110, 116, 117, 122, 124, 125, 126
infectious agents, 117
inflammation, 4, 40, 117, 124, 126
intervention, ix, 33, 49, 116, 120, 121
intracerebral bleed, 48, 50
intracerebral hemorrhage, 36, 57
intracranial pressure, 42, 47
intravenously, ix, 116, 122
ionotropin, 64, 65, 66, 75, 81, 83, 85, 86, 87, 92, 94, 99, 108, 109, 110
ions, 70, 71, 81, 85, 89, 90, 93, 98, 121
ischemia, 35, 36, 41, 45, 46, 117
isolation, ix, 63, 64, 66, 69, 87, 95

K

kidney, 85, 87, 88, 119

L

lesions, ix, 14, 43, 45, 49, 60, 115, 118
leukocytes, 122
leukocytosis, 123
lipid peroxidation, 116
liver, 3, 6, 31
liver function tests, 6
loss of consciousness, 4
low platelet count, 3, 31

M

magnesium, ix, 6, 7, 12, 50, 116, 121
magnetic resonance, 46, 60
magnetic resonance imaging, 46, 60
mammalian cardiotonic steroids, 64, 106
mammals, 66, 77, 80, 82, 83, 84
management, vii, ix, 6, 7, 47, 51, 52, 55, 59, 60, 116, 117, 120, 122, 125, 127
marinobufagenin, 64, 86, 106, 110
measurement, 82, 105, 120
medical, 5, 7, 9, 26, 32, 44, 46, 51
metabolic syndrome, 119
milk, 81, 88, 94
miltefosine, 92, 96, 97, 98
mineralocorticoid, 92
molecular mass, 74
molecular weight, 47
molecules, 67, 73, 75
morbidity, 3, 30, 44, 52, 54, 104, 116
mortality, 3, 30, 44, 47, 52, 59, 104, 116

N

neuroimaging, 7, 13, 17, 33, 44, 46
neurologic symptom, 36
neurological complications, v, vii, 1, 2, 3, 4, 8, 9, 10, 11, 12, 17, 18, 19, 21, 22, 23, 28, 30, 31, 34, 41, 49, 51
nomenclature, 67
normal distribution, 100
nuclear receptor, viii, 63, 87
nutrition, 88, 89, 94, 96

O

obesity, 41, 119, 126
occipital cortex, 45
occipital lobe, 16, 35, 43

oedema, 3, 4, 6, 12, 13, 16, 17, 20, 27, 28, 30, 31, 33, 35, 36, 37, 38, 39, 41, 43, 44, 47, 48
organ, ix, x, 111, 115, 116, 117, 123, 124
orphan disease, 95
ouabain, 64, 65, 66, 69, 82, 83, 87, 89, 105, 106, 108, 110, 113
oxygen, 6, 67, 68, 74, 99
oysters, 82, 109

P

papilledema, 12, 33, 42, 51
paradigm shift, 54, 86
parenchyma, 37, 39, 41, 42, 43
pathogenesis, ix, 36, 56, 95, 116, 117, 118, 119, 124
pathology, ix, 16, 17, 18, 35, 47, 51, 87, 94, 104, 115, 116
pathophysiology, 38, 103
perfusion, 4, 31, 35, 36, 44, 48, 59, 89, 102
pilot study, 101, 104, 107, 112
placenta, 96, 122
platelet activating factor, 74
polymerase chain reaction, 123
population, 37, 41, 47, 93, 100, 120
potassium, viii, 63, 64, 65, 67, 68, 85, 87, 88, 89, 90, 91, 92, 94, 96, 101, 102, 104, 105, 110
potassium sparing diuretics, 64, 89
potassium sparing hormones, viii, 63, 64, 65, 67, 84, 85, 91, 92, 94, 96, 102
pregnancy, vii, viii, ix, 3, 5, 10, 30, 31, 33, 34, 37, 39, 40, 45, 48, 49, 51, 55, 56, 57, 58, 59, 60, 63, 89, 90, 92, 95, 104, 105, 110, 112, 115, 119, 123, 124, 125
preterm delivery, 47
prevention, ix, 6, 47, 50, 51, 60, 112, 116, 118, 119, 120, 121, 125
prognosis, vii, 1, 2, 4, 6, 46, 50, 51

proteinuria, viii, 2, 3, 5, 6, 10, 30, 32, 64, 65, 88, 89, 94, 101, 106, 116, 118, 122
puerperium, ix, 3, 33, 37, 40, 55, 56, 57, 58, 59, 60, 115, 117, 120, 124
P-value, 8, 19, 20, 21, 22, 23, 24, 25, 26
Pxxx, 67

R

recognition, 49, 68, 96
recommendations, iv, 50, 120
recovery, 6, 7, 27, 28, 29, 45, 85, 117, 124, 126
regression, 7, 8, 22, 24, 25, 31, 34, 38, 119
regression analysis, 22, 31, 34, 38
renal failure, 3, 10, 26, 31, 32, 94, 105
reproductive age, 57
requirements, 80, 89
resistance, ix, 116, 123
response, ix, 35, 36, 43, 65, 90, 102, 109, 116
retinal detachment, viii, 2, 5, 10, 12, 26, 27, 28, 32, 33, 44
retinopathy, 12, 21, 33, 46, 55
rhamnose, 66, 108
risk factors, vii, viii, 1, 2, 3, 4, 8, 18, 22, 24, 25, 34, 37, 39, 53, 54, 55, 57, 59, 65, 119, 124, 126, 127

S

sensitivity, 39, 66, 69, 118, 123
sepsis, 41, 118, 123, 124
serum, 65, 66, 68, 69, 70, 71, 80, 81, 82, 83, 87, 89, 90, 92, 93, 94, 95, 97, 98, 99, 102, 103, 104, 106, 111, 121, 122
sexually transmitted diseases, 123
Smith-Lemli-Opitz syndrome (SLO), 68, 81, 85, 87, 88, 107, 108, 109
spiral steroids, viii, 63, 64, 65, 67, 68, 78, 79, 81, 82, 83, 84, 86, 87, 88, 89, 90, 94,

95, 96, 99, 101, 102, 103, 104, 106, 110, 112
steroids, viii, 63, 64, 65, 66, 67, 68, 72, 77, 78, 79, 80, 81, 82, 83, 84, 85, 86, 88, 89, 90, 92, 94, 95, 96, 99, 101, 102, 103, 104, 106, 108, 110, 112, 113
stress, 117, 125
stroke, ix, 3, 4, 5, 36, 37, 38, 39, 40, 43, 46, 47, 49, 50, 53, 54, 55, 56, 57, 58, 59, 60, 94, 105, 116, 120, 127
substrate, 81, 92
sulfate, ix, 61, 87, 116, 121
symptoms, vii, viii, 5, 10, 11, 18, 19, 26, 34, 42, 44, 63, 64, 65, 85, 89, 94, 101, 102, 105, 106
syndrome, viii, ix, 2, 3, 4, 9, 10, 22, 26, 31, 32, 36, 40, 43, 54, 55, 56, 58, 64, 68, 81, 87, 88, 94, 95, 101, 102, 106, 107, 108, 116, 118, 123, 127
synthesis, 80, 81, 85, 92, 94, 101, 104, 106, 117
systolic blood pressure, 18, 34, 50, 54
systolic pressure, 6, 32

T

therapy, ix, 6, 7, 33, 35, 43, 46, 48, 49, 59, 66, 69, 88, 116, 120, 123
thiazide diuretics, 121
thrombolytic therapy, 39
thrombosis, 4, 13, 15, 33, 36, 37, 40, 42, 44, 55, 57, 58, 59, 60
tissue, 36, 41, 47, 82, 87, 96, 118, 121
tissue plasminogen activator, 47
tonic, 3, 5, 30
tonic-clonic seizures, 30
transformation, 40, 109
treatment, 44, 46, 49, 51, 82, 105, 120
trial, 56, 74, 75, 77, 99, 126
trial-and-error, 74, 75, 77, 99

Type 1, 68, 69, 88
Type 2, 68, 88

U

umbilical cord, 93
urea, 122
uric acid, 118
urinalysis, 122
urinary tract, 117
urinary tract infection, 117

V

vascular dementia, 4, 49
vascular system, 42
vasculature, 4, 36
vasoconstriction, 4, 36, 56
vasospasm, 4, 30, 35, 36, 37, 44
vein, 13, 15, 16, 33, 37, 41, 42, 57, 93
vision, 10, 26, 27, 28, 33, 44
visual acuity, 7, 27
visual field, 7, 27
visual field test, 7, 27
visualization, 42
vitamin D, 50, 61
vitamin D deficiency, 50, 61
vomiting, 10, 21, 22

W

weight gain, 94
weight loss, 94
white matter, 13, 14, 16, 38, 49, 60
World Health Organization, 5, 52, 53, 54

Z

Z-scores, 97, 99, 100